Better Breast Health Naturally

with Chinese Medicine

Honora Lee Wolfe & Bob Flaws

BLUE POPPY PRESS

Published by:
BLUE POPPY PRESS, INC.
3450 PENROSE PLACE, SUITE 110
BOULDER, CO 80304

First Edition, January, 1998
ISBN 0-936185-90-2 LC 97-78086
COPYRIGHT 1998 © BLUE POPPY PRESS

COMP Designation: Original work using a standard translational terminology
Printed at Johnson's Printing in Boulder, CO
on essentially chlorine-free paper
Cover design by Jeff Fuller of Crescent Moon
10 9 8 7 6 5 4 3 2 1

Other books in this series include:

Curing Insomnia Naturally with Chinese Medicine
Curing Hay Fever Naturally with Chinese Medicine
Curing Depression Naturally with Chinese Medicine
Curing Arthritis Naturally with Chinese Medicine
Curing PMS Naturally with Chinese Medicine

Preface

In 1989, Blue Poppy Press published my first laywoman's book on Chinese medicine and breast disease titled *The Breast Connection*. During the early '90s, I had the opportunity to make revisions to this first book each time it went into another printing. However, when Blue Poppy's inventories of this perennial good seller became low last year, everyone at Blue Poppy agreed that the book needed more than cosmetic changes.

During 1997, Blue Poppy Press launched a series of laypersons' books on Chinese medicine and various diseases or health concerns. Each of the books in this series shares a common title, cover design, and outline. This series was conceived and designed by Bob Flaws. In particular, he is responsible for the Chinese medical theory and research in each. Therefore, in rewriting this book to fit this series, Bob and I sat down together and coauthored the present text. Bob has spent the last 17 years specializing in Chinese gynecology, and he brings to this edition not only his Chinese medical scholarship but his extensive clinical experience in treating women's breast disease.

In addition, because Western medical science continues to make advances in its understanding and treatment of breast disease, I have changed some of what I say about Western medicine and added new material. Hopefully, Western women will find this book an even more useful resource on the wisdom of Chinese medicine when it comes to diseases of the breasts. Chinese medicine has a great deal of insight into the causes, mechanisms, treatment, and prevention of breast disease which could save many women much suffering and grief were this information more widely known.

Good luck and good health! Sincerely,

Honora Lee Wolfe
January 1, 1998

Table of Contents

Introduction: What's Wrong with This Picture?

From the onset of her period at age 13, Sarah had had severe menstrual cramps and swollen breasts. At age 25 she was diagnosed as having fibrocystic breast disease and severe PMS. The lumpiness was always worse after ovulation and somewhat relieved by the onset of menstruation. When the lumps and pain were at their worst, Sarah didn't even want her husband to hug her, much less make love. As Sarah got older, the lumps got harder and some had to be drained by aspiration. At 38, she had one of the lumps, a benign fibroadenoma, surgically removed. As she approached menopause, other of Sarah's premenstrual symptoms worsened as well. Over the years, Western medicine had offered little help. Research suggests that Sarah is statistically at greater risk for breast cancer because of her fibrocystic breasts.[1] What can be done to help Sarah lower this risk?

Breast diseases are all too common among 20th century American women. More than half of all American women have some medical complaint concerning their breasts at some time during their lives. In a recent article appearing in *The Journal of Chinese Medicine*, Mazin Al-Khafaji states that 45-55% of all Western women will have palpable neoplasms (growths) of the

---

[1] *Macleans*, "Research", April 14, 1997, Vol. 110, #15, p.56. This study included 818 women in Canada with dense, fibrous breast tissue. Results indicated that these women were five times more likely to get breast cancer, and that they were able to reduce their statistical chance of getting cancer by switching to a low fat diet.

breast.[2] Although only a small percentage of these will be life-threatening, such neoplasms can be both painful and frightening, thus affecting other aspects of a woman's life as well.

For most women, breast disease is an even more frightening topic than many other, more often life-threatening diseases, such as heart disease. There are a number of psychological and sociological reasons why this is so. One important reason, however, is that the Western medical treatment of breast diseases is not entirely satisfactory. Western medicine has few if any treatments to offer for so-called benign breast diseases. And, while radical mastectomies have decreased and lumpectomies have increased in recent years for the treatment of breast malignancies, women still fear the surgical invasion and mutilation of their bodies. Many are as frightened of the therapy as of the disease itself. The loss or disfigurement of a breast has an impact on one's psychological and sexual self-image much greater than the actual physical experience.

Chinese medicine, on the other hand, has both a rational and humane theory about the causation and prevention of breast disease as well as effective treatments for most breast diseases. It is especially important for women to understand that, according to Chinese medicine, various diseases of the breast are, in fact, related and have the same or similar disease mechanisms. Because Chinese medicine sees and describe these relationships and can diagnose and effectively treat breast diseases in their early stages, it can help women avoid more serious breast diseases altogether.

For women who have serious breast disease, *i.e.*, who have developed breast cancer, a combination of Western and traditional Chinese medicines is, in many cases, an effective approach.

---

[2]   Al-Khafaji, Mazin, "The Differentiation and Treatment of Mammary Dysplasia and Fibroadenoma by Chinese Medicine," *Journal of Chinese Medicine,* UK, #28, September, 1988.

For the successful story of one woman's treatment using such a combined approach to breast cancer, see Juliet Whitman's *Breast Cancer Journal: A Century of Petals*. (See the annotated bibliography at the back of this book for complete information about this and other books mentioned in the text.) However, if a woman understands the Chinese view concerning the cause and progression of breast disease, she should be much better able to prevent any serious disease from arising in the first place.

This book is an attempt to explain the insights of Chinese medicine concerning breast disease to Western women. It is offered in the hope that it may help alleviate some of the worry, pain, and suffering of women with breast disease by providing them with a clear explanation of their disease, possible preventive measures they may take, and logical treatment alternatives. But before we can appreciate the logic and wisdom of the Chinese medical approach to women's breast disease, we need to know something more about Western medicine and its approach to breast disease.

Western Medicine & Women's Breasts

A ccording to Western anatomy, each breast is composed of 15-25 lobes of glandular tissue which open into the nipple. These lobes are surrounded by fat which give the mass and smooth contour to the breast. Fibrous connective tissue called the Cooper's ligament binds the breast together and provides support and protection for the glandular lobes.

Each lobe contains a duct system of lobules which is capable of conducting milk. The milk is produced by special cells called Acini cells, and transported through the lobules to the nipple. These duct systems are rather like tributaries flowing into a river. These tributaries flow into a main reservoir directly behind the areola, the dark area surrounding the nipple. The milk can then flow from this reservoir to the surface of the nipple via another smaller system of ducts. The breasts are surrounded by lymph nodes which help keep them free from infection. (See Figure 1.)

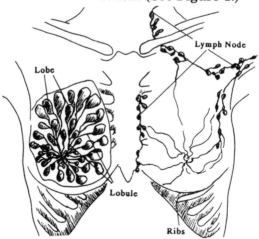

Figure 1.

5

In different women and at different times in even a single woman's life, breast tissue may variously feel soft, like fat tissue, or lumpy and thick, like glandular tissue. Women should get to know what is *normal for them* by doing regular breast self-examination. Every woman should learn how to do and make a routine self-examination of her breasts a non-discretionary part of her life each month. Most gynecologists, Planned Parenthood offices, women's clinics, and cancer research centers have pamphlets or videotapes explaining how to do a proper breast self-examination.

During periods of lactation, which is the sole *biological* function of the breast, the lobes get larger, causing the breasts to expand in size. In most women, the breasts are also highly erogenous and responsive to sexual arousal. There may be changes in the color and texture of the skin of the breast during sexual activity, and the nipples will usually become very erect.

Other changes in the size and texture of the breast tissue during puberty, after the weaning of a child, and during menopause are regulated by the body's endocrine and lymphatic systems. After a period of lactation, the breast may initially shrink to a smaller size than prior to pregnancy, then slowly return to a normal or even a larger size than before. The breast tissue may also be softer than before. During menopause, the instability in the flow of hormones in the body may cause the breasts to increase even more in size. This increase may be temporary or the breasts may remain larger until a woman is very old, at which time the breast tissue becomes flaccid and the size of the breasts again shrinks. These changes are all normal.[3]

---

[3]   Cooper, Patricia, ed., *Better Homes & Gardens Women's Health and Medical Guide*, Meredith Corporation, Publisher, Des Moines, IA, 1981, p.542

1) Premenstrual Breast Distention & Pain

Premenstrual breast distention and pain are two of the most common premenstrual complaints. Premenstrual breast distention and pain are often also a precursor to fibrocystic breast condition. Dr. Niels H. Lauersen, in his book *PMS*, indicates that breast pain and distention are caused by hormonal changes (disturbances in the estrogen/progesterone levels) after ovulation and prior to menstruation each month.[4] Dr. Lauersen states that these changes are considered to be normal in most women. Since it is usually a self-limiting phenomenon related to the menses, it is rarely treated by Western medicine at all. Pain in the breast is not considered to be a common sign of breast cancer, but may be a sign of a breast cyst.[5] Such cysts are usually surgically removed.

2) Fibrocystic Breasts

Fibrocystic changes in the tissue of the breast are the most common of all benign breasts disorders. As many as 30% of all American women may have fibrocystic breasts. This condition usually occurs in women over 25, although new lumps rarely appear in post-menopausal women. Wester medicine holds that fibrocystic breasts are due to a hormonal imbalance. This hormonal imbalance can be triggered by a vast range of causes.[6] No one specific cause has been identified. In this case, estrogen secretion is excessive. This excessive estrogen then stimulates the growth of the glandular lobes and fibrous tissue of the breast, creating many small lumps and distention usually in the outer

---

[4] Lauerson, N.H., & Stukane, E., *PMS: PMS And You*, Simon & Shuster, Inc., NY, 1983, p. 118

[5] Cooper, Patricia, ed., *op. cit.*, p. 546

[6] Berkow, Robert, & Talbott, John, ed., *The Merck Manual of Diagnosis and Therapy*, Merck, Sharp, & Dohme Research Labs, Rahway, NJ, 1977, p. 971

areas of the breast. The major symptom of this condition is visible swelling and pain with palpable lumpiness or thickening in the tissue. The lumps commonly come and go, and the condition is usually worse during the week prior to menstruation.

Because estrogen is relatively excessive in women with fibro-cystic breasts, some Western clinicians refer to this as hyperestrogenonsis (the condition of having too much estrogen). However, there is now debate within the Western medical community whether estrogen secretion is truly excessive or only appears to be so due to a progesterone insufficiency. As women age, the ovaries function less and less perfectly, and a luteal phase defect often goes along with worsening PMS and fibrocystic breasts. The luteal phase is the part of the menstrual cycle from ovulation to the onset of the menses. During this phase, the ovaries main job is to secrete progesterone. If the ovaries fail to secrete enough progesterone, estrogen appears to be excessive, giving rise to a host of pathological changes associated with hyperestrogenosis. (See Figure 2)

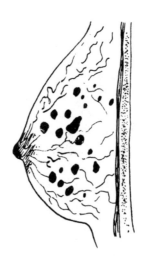

Figure 2.
Fibrocystic Lumps

If fibrocystic breasts are accompanied by fluid-filled lumps, the Western medical treatment of this condition may include aspiration of the larger lumps. This is a procedure usually performed in a doctor's office, whereby a hypodermic needle is inserted directly into the lump to draw out any fluid. It is the only standard Western medical care given to women with fibrocystic breasts. (See Figure 3)

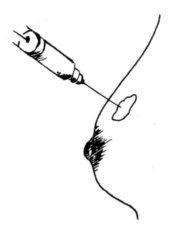

**Figure 3.
Aspiration**

Until recently, fibrocystic breasts were referred to by the acronym FBD, fibrocystic breast *disease*. Recently, Western doctors have decided that fibrocystic changes in the breasts should not be labeled as a disease. Rather, such changes are part of the breasts aging process. As mentioned above, it is now thought that it is the normal aging of the ovaries which causes an estrogen/progesterone imbalance. However, even when Western medicine did label this condition as pathological (*i.e.*, a disease), it had no treatment other than aspiration to offer. Nevertheless, some Western research indicates that women with fibrocystic breast disease are three times more likely to develop breast cancer later in life than those without it.[7] As we will see, below, Chinese medicine does not consider these changes normal and does offer treatment for them, both to stop their progression and *even reverse them*!

3) Fibroadenomas

This is the most common type of tumor seen in younger women and is considered to be the third most frequent of all breast diseases after fibrocystic disease and breast cancer. Fibroadenomas are not malignant. The lump is firm, round, and moveable, like a marble under the skin. According to Western medicine, their cause is unknown. If they are painful or cause breast deformity, they are removed with local anesthesia. In and of itself, fibroadenomas are not considered serious, although their presence indicates the possibility of a higher risk for breast cancer later in life.[8] Chinese medical theory corroborates this increased risk. (See Figure 4)

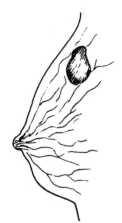

Figure 4.
Fibroadenoma

---

[7] *Ibid.*, p. 971

[8] Cooke, C.W., & Dworkin, S., *op.cit.*, p. 358

If a fibroadenoma or cyst breaks down of its own accord, it can develop into what are called calcifications or microcalcifications. These are grainy calcium deposits developing as a breast cyst breaks down. Microcalcifications may or may not be associated with the development of breast cancer.

4) Breast Abscesses (Mastitis)

Due to local or systemic infection in the glands and ducts of the breast, this condition manifests as a painful, inflamed mass sometimes accompanied by discharge from the nipple. It is most commonly experienced after childbirth and during breast feeding, usually in a primapara (first time mother). When treated by Western medicine, breast feeding is often stopped and surgical drainage and/or antibiotics are administered.[9]

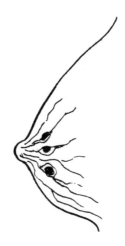

Figure 5.
Intraductal Papilloma

---

[9] Berkow, R., & Talbott, J., *op. cit.*, p. 970

5) Intraductal Papillomas

These are very small tumors occurring in the terminal nipple ducts of the breast. They are frequently so small they are impossible to palpate. The main symptom is a serous, pinkish, or bloody discharge from the nipple. Treatment consists of surgical removal of the affected ducts and any other affected part of the breast. According to Western medicine, this tissue must be biopsied since a bloody discharge from the nipple can be due to malignancy especially if it occurs in only one breast.[10] (See Figure 5.)

6) Breast Cancer

Cancer of the breast is second only to lung cancer in deadliness and to skin cancers in frequency of occurrence in women, accounting for one out of every three cancers diagnosed in women. The American Cancer Society estimates that in 1996, 184,300 new cases of this disease were diagnosed in the U.S. and that 44,300 women died of it.[11] Approximately one woman in eight in this country will develop breast cancer at some point in her life at its present rate of occurrence. This is an increase from one in 10 since 1988. Carcinoma of the breast is the most common of all breast malignancies and carries with it the highest rate of mortality.[12] Signs of this disease include 1) a lump or thickening in the breast or armpit, 2) a change in the size or shape of the breast, 3) a bloody, brown, or green discharge from the nipple, and/or 4) a change in the color or texture of the skin of the breast or areola, such as dimpling, puckering, or scaliness. Pain is rarely an early sign of breast cancer. According to

---

[10] *Ibid.*, p .972

[11] American Cancer Society Surveillance Research Bulletin, 1996 *Breast Cancer: Facts and Figures*, 1996

[12] Berkow, R., & Talbott, J. *op. cit.*, p. 972

Western medicine, the earlier breast cancer is detected and treated, the better are a woman's chance of complete recovery.

Western medical diagnosis of breast cancer is usually made by a combination of palpation (feeling the size, texture, and movability of a lump or thickening), aspiration (using a needle and syringe to withdraw fluid or tissue for biopsy), mammography (breast x-ray to reveal tumors which cannot be felt), and biopsy (removal of some or all of the lump to check for cancerous cells). Other tests such as ultrasonography or thermography may also be used.

Depending upon what stage of cancer is discovered, Western medical treatment may include lumpectomy, simple or radical mastectomy, chemotherapy, radiation therapy, or hormone therapy. Most treatment involves two or more of these, done in stages.[13]

According to Western medicine, the cause of breast cancer is unknown but some women seem to have higher risk than others for developing the disease. Factors include:

1. Age. The incidence of breast cancer increases in women as they age. In fact, it is now believed in some epidemiology circles that all women, if they live long enough, will eventually develop breast cancer, just as all men, if they live long enough, will also develop prostate cancer. Since not all breast cancers are fast growing, many elderly women die of other causes, never knowing that they harbored cancerous cells in their breasts. We will discuss what Chinese medicine has to say about this at length below.

2. Family history. The risk doubles if a mother, daughter, or sister has had the disease.

---

[13] Anon., *What You Need To Know About Breast Cancer*, U.S. Department of Health & Human Services, 1988, p. 10-11

3. Personal history. A history of benign breast cysts, early onset of menstruation, late or no childbirths, or late menopause are all associated with an increased risk of developing breast cancer.[14]

Recent Western research indicates that diet may also affect the chances of contracting some types of cancer. Breast cancer appears to be more likely to occur in women whose diet is high in fat, low in fiber, and who are generally overweight.[15]

Whatever the causes, *any* woman can get breast cancer and *all* women should do breast self-examination every month[16], get regular health check-ups, and see a primary health care practitioner if any abnormal changes occur.

The Shortcomings of Western Medicine When It Comes to Breast Disease

Western medicine is physical medicine. It describes in great detail the material structure and interrelationships of the tissues, cells, and chemical constituents of the human body. Its treatments tend to be swift, heroic, and invasive. While this type of therapy has its strong points and can be miraculous, it often causes unwanted side effects. Furthermore, it rarely deals with the root causes of disease. Because Western medicine typically fails to identify and address the root cause of so many diseases, it offers little to patients in terms of preventive measures.

---

[14] *Ibid.*, p. 22-23

[15] Shell, E.R., *op. cit.*, p.246

[16] For information on the most effective way to do a breast self-exam, see the section on self-help and home remedies later in this book.

14

For most of the breast diseases described above, the only Western medical therapy available is removal of palpable lumps by surgery or aspiration. Few preventive measures are offered and, for some disorders, there is no Western medical treatment. This is so despite the fact that some Western medical research indicates a higher incidence of breast cancer in women who have had other breast diseases. Western medicine finds no rational, theoretical link between one breast disease entity and another.

Chinese medicine, on the other hand, sees breast diseases as a continuum from premenstrual breast disease through fibrocystic breasts to breast cancer. Based on its holistic vision of the cause and mechanisms of breast disease, Chinese medicine offers both remedial treatment for all breast diseases as well as, and perhaps even more importantly, numerous self-help techniques for preventing breast disease altogether.

The Differences Between Modern Western & Traditional Chinese Medicine

In order for the reader to understand and make sense of the rest of this book on Chinese medicine and women's breast disease, one must understand that Chinese medicine is a distinct and separate system of medical thought and practice from modern Western medicine. This means that one must shift models of reality when it comes to thinking about Chinese medicine. It has taken the Chinese more than 2,000 years to develop this medical system. In fact, Chinese medicine is the oldest continually practiced, literate, professional medicine in the world. As such one cannot understand Chinese medicine by trying to explain it in Western scientific or medical terms.

Most people reading this book have probably taken high school biology back when they were sophomores. Whether we recognize it or not, most of us Westerners think of what we learned about the human body in high school as "the really real" description of reality, not one possible description. However, if Chinese medicine is to make any sense to Westerners at all, one must be able to entertain the notion that there are potentially other valid descriptions of the human body, its functions, health, and disease. In grappling with this fundamentally important issue, it is useful to think about the concepts of a map and the terrain it describes.

If we take the United States of America as an example, we can have numerous different maps of this country's land mass. One map might show population. Another might show per capita incomes. Another might show religious or ethnic distributions. Yet another might be a road map. And still another might be a map showing political, *i.e.*, state boundaries. In fact, there could be an infinite number of potentially different maps of the United States depending on what one was trying to show and do. As long as the map is based on accurate information and has been created with self-consistent logic, then one map is not necessarily more correct than another. The issue is to use the right map for what you are trying to do. If one wants to drive from Chicago to Washington, D.C., then a road map is probably the right one for that job but is not necessarily a truer or "more real" description of the United States than a map showing annual rainfall.

What we are getting at here is that the map is not the terrain. The Western biological map of the human body is only one potentially useful medical map. It is no more true than the traditional Chinese medical map, and the "facts" of one map cannot be reduced to the criteria or standards of another unless they share the same logic right from the beginning. As long as the Western medical map is capable of solving a person's disease in a cost-effective, time-efficient manner without side effects or iatrogenesis (meaning doctor-caused disease), then it is a useful map. Chinese medicine needs to be judged in the same way. The Chinese medical map of health and disease is just as "real" as the Western biological map as long as using it professional practitioners and their patients are able to solve their patients' health problems in a safe and effective way.

The following chapter is an introduction to the basics of Chinese medicine. Unless one understands some of the fundamental theories and "facts" of Chinese medicine, one will not be able to understand or accept the reasons for some of the Chinese medical treatments of breast disease. As the reader will quickly see from this brief overview of Chinese medicine, "This doesn't look like Kansas, Toto!"

An Overview of the Chinese Medical Map

In this chapter, we will look at an overview of Chinese medicine. In particular, we will discuss yin and yang, qi, blood, and essence, the viscera and bowels, and the channels and network vessels. Then, in the following chapters, we will go on to see how Chinese medicine views the menstrual cycle and the mechanisms at work in breast disease. After that, we will look at the Chinese medical diagnosis and treatment of breast diseases.

Yin & Yang

To understand Chinese medicine, one must first understand the concepts of yin and yang since these are the most basic concepts in this system. Yin and yang are the cornerstones for understanding, diagnosing, and treating the body and mind in Chinese medicine. In a sense, all the other theories and concepts of Chinese medicine are nothing other than an elaboration of yin and yang. Most people have probably already heard of yin and yang but may have only a fuzzy idea of what these terms mean.

The concepts of yin and yang can be used to describe everything that exists in the universe, including all the parts and functions of the body. Originally, yin referred to the shady side of a hill and yang to the sunny side of the hill. Since sunshine and shade are two, interdependent sides of a single reality, these two aspects of the hill are seen as part of a single whole. Other examples of yin and yang are that night exists only in relation to day and cold exists only in relation to heat. According to Chinese thought, every single thing that exists in the universe has these two aspects, a yin and a yang. Thus everything has a front and a back, a top and a bottom, a left and a right, and a beginning and an end. However, a thing is yin or yang *only in relation to its paired complement.* Nothing is in itself yin or yang.

It is the concepts of yin and yang which make Chinese medicine a holistic medicine. This is because, based on this unitary and complementary vision of reality, no body part or body function is viewed as separate or isolated from the whole person. The table below shows a partial list of yin and yang pairs as they apply to

Yin	Yang
form	function
organs	bowels
blood	qi
inside	outside
front of body	back of body
right side	left side
lower body	upper body
cool, cold	warm, hot
stillness	activity, movement

the body. However, it is important to remember that each item listed is either yin or yang only in relation to its complementary partner. Nothing is absolutely and all by itself either yin or yang. As we can see from the above list, it is possible to describe every aspect of the body in terms of yin and yang.

Qi

Qi (pronounced chee) and blood are the two most important complementary pairs of yin and yang within the human body. It is said that, in the world, yin and yang are water and fire, but in the human body, yin and yang are blood and qi. Qi is yang in relation to blood which is yin. Qi is often translated as energy and certainly energy is a manifestation of qi. Chinese language scholars would say, however, that qi is larger than any single type of energy described by modern Western science. Paul Unschuld, perhaps the greatest living sinologist, translates the word qi as influences. This conveys the sense that qi is what is responsible for change and movement. Thus, within Chinese medicine, qi is that which motivates all movement and transformation or change.

In Chinese medicine, qi is defined as having five specific functions:

1. Defense

It is qi which is responsible for protecting the exterior of the body from invasion by external pathogens. This qi, called defensive qi, flows through the exterior portion of the body.

2. Transformation

Qi transforms substances so that they can be utilized by the body. An example of this function is the transformation of the food we eat into nutrients to nourish the body, thus producing more qi and blood.

3. Warming

Qi, being relatively yang, is inherently warm and one of the main functions of the qi is to warm the entire body, both inside and out. If this warming function of the qi is weak, cold may cause the flow of qi and blood to be congealed similar to cold's effect on water producing ice.

4. Restraint

It is qi which holds all the organs and substances in their proper place. Thus all the organs, blood, and fluids need qi to keep them from falling or leaking out of their specific pathways. If this function of the qi is weak, then problems like uterine prolapse, easy bruising, or urinary incontinence may occur.

5. Transportation

Qi provides the motivating force for all transportation and movement in the body. Every aspect of the body that moves is moved by the qi. Hence the qi moves the blood and body fluids throughout the body. It moves food through the stomach and blood through the vessels.

Blood

In Chinese medicine, blood refers to the red fluid that flows through our vessels the same as in modern Western medicine, but it also has meanings and implications which are different from those in modern Western medicine. Most basically, blood is that substance which nourishes and moistens all the body tissues. Without blood, no body tissue can function properly. In addition, when blood is insufficient or scanty, tissue becomes dry and withers.

Qi and blood are closely interrelated. It is said that, "Qi is the commander of the blood and blood is the mother of qi." This means that it is qi which moves the blood but that it is the blood which provides the nourishment and physical foundation for the creation and existence of the qi.

In Chinese medicine, blood provides the following functions for the body:

1. Nourishment

Blood nourishes the body. Along with qi, the blood goes to every part of the body. When the blood is insufficient, function decreases and tissue atrophies or shrinks.

2. Moistening

Blood moistens the body tissues. This includes the skin, eyes, and ligaments and tendons or what are simply called the sinews of the body in Chinese medicine. Thus blood insufficiency can cause drying out and consequent stiffening of various body tissues throughout the body.

3. Blood provides the material foundation for the spirit or mind.

In Chinese medicine, the mind and body are not two separate things. The spirit is nothing other than a great accumulation of qi. The blood (yin) supplies the material support and nourishment for the spirit (yang) so that it accumulates, becomes bright (i.e., conscious and clever), and stays rooted in the body. If the blood becomes insufficient, the mind can "float," causing problems like insomnia, agitation, and unrest.

Essence

Along with qi and blood, essence is one of the three most important constituents of the body. Essence is the most fundamental, essential material the body utilizes for its growth, maturation, and reproduction. There are two forms of this essence. We inherit essence from our parents and we also produce our own essence from the food we eat, the liquids we drink, and the air we breathe.

The essence which comes from our parents is what determines our basic constitution, strength, and vitality. We each have a finite, limited amount of this inherited essence. It is important to protect and conserve this essence because all bodily functions depend upon it, and, when it is gone, we die. Thus the depletion of essence has serious implications for our overall health and well-being. Happily, the essence derived from food and drink helps to bolster and support this inherited essence. Thus, if we eat well and do not consume more qi and blood than we create each day, then when we sleep at night, this surplus qi and more especially blood is transformed into essence.

The Viscera & Bowels

In Chinese medicine, the internal organs (called viscera so as not to become confused with the Western biological entities of the same name) have a wider area of function and influence than in Western medicine. Each viscus has distinct responsibilities for maintaining the physical and psychological health of the individual. When thinking about the internal viscera according to Chinese medicine, it is more accurate to view them as spheres of influence or as zones of greatly concentrated energetic activity which spread throughout the larger energetic grid or template of the body[17] rather than as a distinct and separate physical organs as described by Western science. This is why the famous German sinologist, Manfred Porkert, refers to them as orbs rather than as organs. In Chinese medicine, each viscus is responsible for a variety of functions which, in relationship to each other, keep the body healthy and in balance. The relationship between the various viscera and other parts of the body is made possible by the channel and network vessel system which we will discuss below.

---

[17] Larre, Claude, Schatz, Jean, & Rochat de la Valle, Elizabeth, *Survey of Traditional Chinese Medicine*, Institut Ricci, Paris, 1986

In Chinese medicine, there are five main viscera which are relatively yin and six main bowels which are relatively yang. The five yin viscera are the heart, lungs, liver, spleen, and kidneys. The six yang bowels are the stomach, small intestine, large intestine, gallbladder, urinary bladder, and a system that Chinese medicine refers to as the triple burner. All the functions of the entire body are subsumed or described under these eleven organs or spheres of influence. Thus Chinese medicine *as a system* does not have a pancreas, a pituitary gland, or the ovaries. Nonetheless, all the functions of these Western organs are described under the Chinese medical system of the five viscera and six bowels.

Within this system, the five viscera are the most important. These are the organs that Chinese medicine says are responsible for the creation and transformation of qi and blood and the storage of essence. For instance, the kidneys are responsible for the excretion of urine but are also responsible for hearing, the strength of the bones, sex, reproduction, maturation and growth, the lower and upper back, and the lower legs in general and the knees in particular.

Visceral Correspondences

Organ	Tissue	Sense	Spirit	Emotion
Kidneys	bones/ head hair	hearing	will	fear
Liver	sinews	sight	ethereal soul	anger
Spleen	flesh	taste	thought	thinking/ worry
Lungs	skin/ body hair	smell	corporeal soul	grief/ sadness
Heart	blood vessels	speech	spirit	joy/ fright

This points out that the Chinese viscera may have the same name and even some overlapping functions but yet are quite different from the organs of modern Western medicine.[18] Each of the five Chinese medical viscera also has a corresponding tissue, sense, spirit, and emotion related to it. These are outlined in the table above.

In addition, each Chinese medical viscus or bowel possesses both a yin and a yang aspect. The yin aspect of a viscus or bowel refers to its substantial nature or tangible form. Further, an organ's yin is responsible for the nurturing, cooling, and moistening of that viscus or bowel. The yang aspect of the viscus or bowel represents its functional activities or what it does. An organ's yang aspect is also warming. These two aspects, yin and yang, form and function, cooling and heating, when balanced create good health. However, if either yin or yang becomes too strong or too weak, the result will be disease.

According to Chinese medical theory, breast diseases, both benign and malignant, are primarily associated with imbalances in three viscera. The liver, spleen, and kidneys. In order to understand the logic of Chinese medicine *vis à vis* breast disease, we must first understand the main Chinese statements of fact concerning these three viscera. They are as follows:

The kidneys

In Chinese medicine, the kidneys are considered to be the foundation of our life. Therefore, we will discuss them first. Because the developing fetus looks like a large kidney and

---

[18] Because the *Chinese* medical definitions of the viscera is functional and energetic, as opposed to strictly material, the authors discourage readers from purchasing any over the counter medicines described as being good for conditions of the *Western* organs. If any reader feels that they have an imbalance in a viscus similar to what is described in this book for which they desire treatment, we suggest that they seek out a professional practitioner of Traditional Chinese Medicine.

because the kidneys are the main viscus for the storage of inherited essence, the kidneys are referred to as the prenatal root. Keeping the kidney qi strong and kidney yin and yang in relative balance is considered essential to good health and longevity. The basic Chinese medical statements of fact about the kidneys are:

1. The kidneys are considered responsible for human reproduction, development, and maturation.

These are the same functions we used when describing the essence. This is because the essence is stored in the kidneys. Health problems related to reproduction, development, and maturation are considered to be problems of the kidney essence. Excessive sexual activity, drug use, or simple prolonged over-exhaustion can all damage and consume kidney essence. Kidney essence is also consumed by the simple act of aging.

2. The kidneys are the foundation of water metabolism.

The kidneys work in coordination with the lungs and spleen to insure that water is spread properly throughout the body and that excess water is excreted as urination. Therefore, problems such as edema, excessive dryness, or excessive day or nighttime urination can indicate a weakness of kidney function.

3. The kidneys are responsible for hearing since the kidneys open through the portals of the ears.

Therefore, auditory problems such as diminished hearing and ringing in the ears can be due to kidney weakness.

5. The kidneys rule the grasping of qi.

This means that one of the functions of the kidney qi is to pull down or absorb the breath from the lungs and root it in the lower abdomen. Certain types of asthma and chronic cough are the result of a weakness in this kidney function.

6. The kidneys rule the bones and marrow.

This means that problems of the bones, such as osteoporosis, degenerative disc disease, and weak legs and knees, can all reflect a kidney problem.

7. Kidney yin and yang are the foundation for the yin and yang of all the other organs and bowels and body tissues of the entire body.

This is another way of saying that the kidneys are the foundation of our life. If either kidney yin or yang is insufficient, eventually the yin or yang of the other organs will also become insufficient.

8. The kidneys store the will.

If kidney qi is insufficient, this aspect of our human nature can be weakened. Conversely, pushing ourselves to extremes, such as long distance running or cycling, can eventually exhaust our kidneys.

9. Fear is the emotion associated with the kidneys.

This means that fear can manifest when the kidney qi is insufficient. Vice versa, constant or excessive fear can damage the kidneys and make them weak.

10. The low back is the mansion of the kidneys.

This means that, of all the areas of the body, the low back is the most closely related to the health of the kidneys. If the kidneys are weak, then there may be low back pain. It is because of this and the fact that the kidneys are associated with the bones that the kidneys are the first and most important viscus in terms of the health and well-being of the low back according to Chinese medicine.

The liver

In Chinese medicine, the liver is associated with one's emotional state, with digestion, and with menstruation in women. As we will see in the following chapters, the liver is the lynchpin in the Chinese medical diagnosis and treatment of breast disease. The basic Chinese medical statements of facts concerning the liver include:

1. The liver controls coursing and discharge.

Coursing and discharge refer to the uninhibited spreading of qi to every part of the body. If the liver is not able to maintain the free and smooth flow of qi throughout the body, multiple physical and emotional symptoms can develop. This function of the liver is most easily damaged by emotional causes and, in particular, by anger and frustration. For example, if the liver is stressed due to pent-up anger, the flow of liver qi can become depressed or stagnate.

If this happens, liver qi stagnation can lead to or worsen a wide range of health problems, including most symptoms of PMS, abdominal and breast pain and distention, chronic digestive disturbance, depression, and low back pain. Therefore, it is essential to keep our liver qi flowing freely.

2. The liver stores the blood.

This means that the liver regulates the amount of blood in circulation. In particular, when the body is at rest, the blood in the extremities returns to the liver. As an extension of this, it is said in Chinese medicine that the liver is yin in form but yang in function. Thus the liver requires sufficient blood to keep it *and its associated tissues* moist and supple, cool and relaxed.

29

3. The liver controls the sinews.

The sinews refer mainly to the tendons and ligaments in the body. Proper function of the tendons and ligaments depends upon the nourishment of liver blood to keep them moist and supple.

4. The liver opens into the portals of the eyes.

The eyes are the specific sense organ corresponding to the liver. Therefore, many eye problems are related to the liver in Chinese medicine.

5. The emotion associated with the liver is anger.

Anger is the emotion that typically arises when the liver is diseased and especially when its qi does not flow freely. Conversely, anger damages the liver. Thus the emotions related to the stagnation of qi in the liver are frustration, anger, and rage.

The spleen

The spleen is less important in Western medicine than it is in Chinese medicine. Since at least the Yuan dynasty (1280-1368 CE), the spleen has been one of the two most important viscera of Chinese medicine (the other being the kidneys). In Chinese medicine, the spleen plays a pivotal role in the creation of qi and blood and in the circulation and transformation of body fluids. Therefore, when it comes to the spleen, it is especially important not to think of this Chinese viscus in the same way as the Western spleen. The spleen plays a vital role in the health of the breasts. The main statements of fact concerning the spleen in Chinese medicine are:

1. The spleen governs movement and transformation.

This refers to the movement and transformation of foods and liquids through the digestive system. In this case, movement and transformation may be paraphrased as digestion. However, secondarily, movement and transformation also refer to the movement and transformation of body fluids through the body. It is the spleen qi which is largely responsible for controlling liquid metabolism in the body.

2. The spleen restrains the blood.

As mentioned above, one of the five functions of the qi is to restrain the fluids of the body, including the blood, within their proper channels and reservoirs. If the spleen qi is healthy and abundant, then the blood is held within its vessels properly. However, if the spleen qi becomes weak and insufficient, then the blood may flow outside its channels and vessels resulting in various types of pathological bleeding. This includes various types of pathological bleeding associated with the menstrual cycle.

3. The spleen stores the constructive.

The constructive is one of the types of qi in the body. Specifically, it is the qi responsible for nourishing and constructing the body and its tissues. This constructive qi is closely associated with the process of digestion and the creation of qi and blood out of food and liquids. If the spleen fails to store or runs out of constructive qi, then the person becomes hungry on the one hand, and eventually becomes fatigued on the other.

4. The spleen governs the muscles and flesh.

This statement is closely allied to the previous one. It is the constructive qi which constructs or nourishes the muscles and flesh. If there is sufficient spleen qi producing sufficient constructive qi, then the person's body is well fleshed and rounded. In addition, their muscles are normally strong. Conversely, if the spleen becomes weak, this may lead to emaciation and/or lack of strength.

5. The spleen governs the four limbs.

This means that the strength and function of the four limbs is closely associated with the spleen. If the spleen is healthy and strong, then there is sufficient strength in the four limbs and warmth in the four extremities. If the spleen becomes weak and insufficient, then there may be lack of strength in the four limbs, lack of warmth in the extremities, or even tingling and numbness in the extremities.

6. The spleen opens into the portal of the mouth.

Just as the ears are the portals of the kidneys, the eyes are the portal of the liver, and the tongue is the portal of the heart, the mouth is the portal of the spleen. Therefore, spleen disease often manifests as mouth or canker sores or bleeding from the gums.

7. Thought is the emotion associated with the spleen.

In the West, we do not usually think of thought as an emotion per se. Be that as it may, in Chinese medicine it is classified along with anger, joy, fear, fright, grief, and melancholy. In particular, thinking, or perhaps I should say overthinking, causes the spleen qi to bind. This means that the spleen qi does not flow harmoniously and this typically manifests as loss of appetite, abdominal bloating after meals, and indigestion.

8. The spleen is the source of engenderment and transformation.

Engenderment and transformation refer to the creation or production of the qi and blood out of the food and drink we take in each day. If the spleen receives adequate food and drink and then properly transforms that food and drink, it engenders or creates the qi and blood. Although the kidneys and lungs also participate in the creation of the qi, while the kidneys and heart also participate in the creation of the blood, the spleen is the pivotal viscus in both processes, and spleen qi weakness and

32

insufficiency is a leading cause of qi and blood insufficiency and weakness.

Because the viscera are relatively more important than the bowels in Chinese medicine, we will not take up the space here to enumerate all the functions of each bowel. Suffice it to say that each viscus is paired with a bowel in a yin-yang relationship. The kidneys are paired with the urinary bladder, the liver is paired with the gallbladder, the heart is paired with the small intestine, the spleen is paired with the stomach, and the lungs are paired with the large intestine. In the case of the urinary bladder, gallbladder, and stomach, these bowels receive their qi from their paired viscus and function very much as an extension of that viscus. The relationship between the other two viscera and bowels is not as close.

Above we mentioned that there are five viscera and six bowels. The sixth bowel is called the triple burner. It is said in Chinese that, "The triple burner has a function but no form." The name triple burner refers to the three main areas of the torso. The upper burner is the chest. The middle burner is the space from the bottom of the rib cage to the level of the navel. The lower burner is the lower abdomen below the navel. These three spaces are called burners because all of the functions and transformations of the viscera and bowels which they contain are "warm" transformations similar to food cooking in a pot on a stove or similar to an alchemical transformation in a furnace. In fact, the triple burner is nothing other than a generalized concept of how the other viscera and bowels function together as an organic unit in terms of the digestion of foods and liquids and the circulation and transformation of body fluids.

For a complete description of all the viscera and bowels, the interested reader should see Ted Kaptchuk's *The Web That Has No Weaver*.

The Channels & Network Vessels

Each viscus and bowel has a corresponding channel with which it is connected. In Chinese medicine, the inside of the body is made up of the viscera and bowels. The outside of the body is composed of the sinews and bones, muscles and flesh, and skin and hair. It is the channels and network vessels (*i.e.*, smaller connecting vessels) which connect the inside and the outside of the body. It is through these channels and network vessels that the viscera and bowels connect with their corresponding body tissues.

The channels and network vessel system is a unique feature of traditional Chinese medicine. These channels and vessels are different from the circulatory, nervous, or lymphatic systems. The earliest reference to these channels and vessels is in *Nei Jing (Inner Classic)*, a text written around the 2nd or 3rd century BCE.

The channels and vessels perform two basic functions. They are the pathways by which the qi and blood circulate through the body and between the organs and tissues. Additionally, as mentioned above, the channels connect the viscera and bowels internally with the exterior part of the body. This channel and vessel system functions in the body much like the world information communication network. The channels allow the various parts of our body to cooperate and interact to maintain our lives.

This channel and network vessel system is complex. There are 12 primary channels, six yin and six yang, each with a specific pathway through the external body and connected with an internal organ (see diagram below). There are also extraordinary vessels, sinew channels, channel divergences, main network vessels, and ultimately countless finer and finer network vessels permeating the entire body. All of these form a closed loop or circuit similar to but distinct from the Western circulatory system.

We will refer to various of these channels as they pertain to the breasts later on in several sections of this book.

34

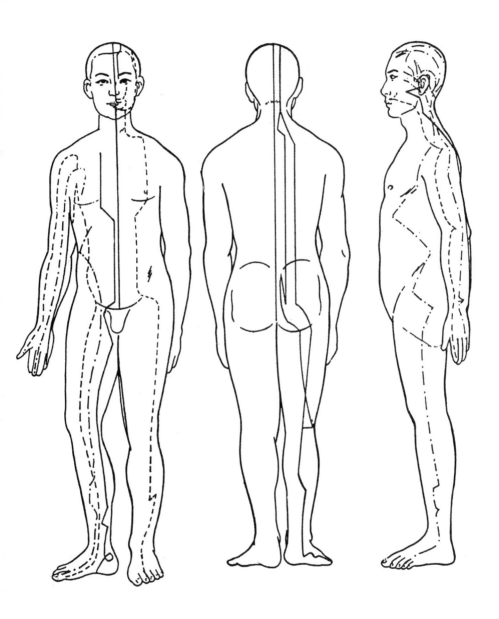

The Menstrual Cycle in Chinese Medicine

In the preceding chapter we discussed the most important of the five viscera and six bowels in terms of breast disease. However, there are in Chinese medicine another set of six "extraordinary bowels" which includes the uterus. It is said in Chinese medicine that men and women are basically the same. However, women have a uterus and thus they menstruate, can conceive, give birth, and lactate. Notice that we said, because women have a uterus, they lactate. A famous saying in Chinese medicine states, "The blood descends and becomes the menstruate; it ascends and becomes the milk." This mean that what happens in the breasts is very much related to what's happening in the uterus. Therefore, before one can understand breast disease, we must take into account the menstrual cycle.

The menses themselves are a discharge of blood. For this discharge to take place, two things have to occur. First, a super-abundance of blood must accumulate in the uterus for it to eventually spill over as the menstruate. And secondly, the qi and blood must be freely and uninhibitedly flowing in order to allow this brimming over. This means that, in order to understand menstruation, one must understand how blood is created and what might affect the free and uninhibited flow of qi and blood.

The creation of blood

There are three viscera which participate in the creation of the blood. These are the kidneys, spleen, and heart. The heart is the place where the blood is "turned red" or finally created. However, first the spleen must send up the finest essence of food and liquids extracted in the process of digestion. If the spleen does not send up this finest essence of food and liquids there will be insufficient supplies for the heart to transform these into blood. In addition, the kidneys must send up some essence to also participate in the creation of blood. One can think of this as somewhat similar to adding some sour dough starter in order to make a new batch of sour dough bread.

In other words, if the kidney lacks sufficient essence, if the spleen fails to digest the finest essence of food and liquids and send this upward, and if the heart, for any reason, cannot fulfill its function of "turning the blood red", then there may be insufficient creation of blood. In addition, it is the heart's job to spread the blood to the rest of the body and eventually move it down to the uterus. It is said in Chinese medicine that first the blood goes to nourish and moisten the viscera and bowels. Then it goes into the channels and vessels. From there it nourishes and moistens the rest of the tissues of the body, and what collects in the uterus is what is left over after the blood has performed all these other jobs. When enough blood collects in the uterus to fill it, it overflows as the menses. Typically, a young to middle-aged, healthy woman will produce such a superabundance accumulating in the uterus once every 28-30 days.

The control of the blood

Although normal menstruation cannot occur if there is insufficient blood accumulated in the uterus, it can occur either too early or too late if the flow of blood is not controlled properly. Just as there are three viscera which engender and transform the blood, there are three viscera which govern or control the blood. These are the heart, liver, and spleen. It is said that the heart qi governs the blood. Above we have seen that this means that it is the heart qi which "stirs" or pushes the blood. If the heart qi does not move the blood, the blood cannot move on its own. Thus it is said:

> The qi moves the blood. If the qi moves, the blood moves. If the qi stops, the blood stops.

38

In actual fact, the heart gets its qi primarily from the spleen. So a sufficiency of spleen qi is necessary for there to be enough heart qi to move the blood. In addition, the spleen qi restrains and contains the blood within its channels and vessels. If the spleen qi is too weak, it may allow the blood to seep out prematurely or it may not cut off menstruation when it should. And finally, the liver stores the blood. It is the liver's job to regulate the amount of blood in circulation. It is the liver qi which performs this function. If the liver qi spreads freely, then the blood moves. If the liver qi becomes depressed and stagnant, then the blood will also eventually become depressed and static.

One may find it hard at first to distinguish the difference between the spleen and the liver's role in maintaining the free and uninhibited flow of blood. It is the spleen qi ultimately (via the heart) which provides the motivating force behind the propulsion of the blood. It is the liver which allows the blood to flow freely through its channels and vessels. If, for instance, one has gas in their car and the car is in good working order, one may have the power to move one's car. However, if one is stopped at a red light, one may not have the permission to move the car even though the power is there. In terms of the heart, spleen and liver, the flow of blood is the same. The heart and spleen provide the motivating power, but it is the liver qi which allows that blood to flow freely or not.

If, for any reason, one of these three viscera does not function correctly in terms of the flow of blood, this may impede the free and timely flow of the menstruate. Since the uterus and the menstruation are linked with the function of the breast, any abnormalities in the function of the three viscera associated with menstruation may also cause abnormal changes in the breast as well.

The four phases of the menstrual cycle

Chinese gynecologists divide the menstrual cycle into four, roughly seven day periods. Phase one begins the day the menses end. If one counts the days of the menstrual cycle from the first day of the onset of menstruation, this means that phase one typically begins on day four, five, six, or seven. The uterus had discharged its accumulated blood and this leaves the body relatively empty or vacuous of blood. Because blood is created, at least in part out of kidney essence and because, compared to yang qi, essence is a type of yin substance, during phase one, the body busies itself with making more yin and blood to replenish that which was discharged. Therefore, in Chinese gynecology, we say that phase one corresponds to yin and the emphasis in the body is on replenishing yin blood.

Phase two corresponds to the days surrounding ovulation. Up till now, the body has been replenishing its yin. However, for ovulation to occur, yin must transform into yang. This transformation of yin into yang corresponds to the rise in basal body temperature which occurs after ovulation.[19] If there is insufficient yin, it cannot transform into yang. Conversely, if there is insufficient yang, it cannot transform yin. In addition, if either the qi and blood are not flowing freely, this transformation may also be impeded. Generally, phase two corresponds to days 10-16 in the monthly cycle and it corresponds to yang in the same way that phase one corresponds to yin.

Phase three corresponds to the premenstruum and to the qi. For things to go as they should in the woman's body, yang qi must stay strong enough long enough and the qi must flow freely and in the right directions. Many of the signs and symptoms of PMS, including premenstrual breast distention and pain, have to do with the yang qi not being strong enough or the qi (and therefore the blood) not flowing freely. Phase three may be counted from day 17 to the day before menstruation, *i.e.*, day 28, and corresponds to qi.

---

[19] Basal body temperature refers to one's resting temperature when taken the first thing upon waking in the morning before getting up, dressing, eating, or doing anything else. It is analogous to one's resting pulse or one's basal metabolic rate. Plotting one's basal body temperature on a graph is one way of determining if and when a woman is ovulating.

40

Phase four is the menstruation itself. Since the onset of menstruation is counted as day one in the cycle, phase four may last anywhere from one or two days to six or seven depending on the individual woman's constitution and age. Because menstruation is a downward discharge of blood according to Chinese medicine, phase four corresponds to the blood.

When looked at from this perspective, the menstrual cycle is made up of four (not always equal) segments corresponding to yin, yang, qi and blood. This relationship is shown in the chart below.

Problems may occur in any of these four phases and may occur for reasons other than the dominant correspondence in that phase. However, when a problem occurs in any of these four phases, the Chinese doctor will first investigate to see if the dominant correspondence, whether yin, yang, qi, or blood, is behaving as it should at that time. *Since PMS occurs in the premenstruum or phase three, most premenstrual complaints, including premenstrual breast distention and pain and fibrocystic breasts, are attributed, either directly or indirectly, to problems with the flow of qi.*

Qi, Blood, Yin & Yang
vis-a-vis Menstrual Cycle

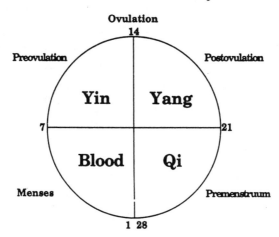

41

Age and the menstrual cycle

In Chinese medicine, the doctor takes everything about the patient into account. This includes their bodily constitution, their temperament, their lifestyle and occupation, and their age. There is a famous saying in Chinese gynecology which runs:

> In adolescent (girls), blame the kidneys.
> In middle-aged (women), blame the liver.
> In older (women), blame the spleen.

When adolescent girls first begin menstruating, their cycles are often irregular. They may go several months or more between menses and their periods may not come regularly every 28-30 until several years after menarche or the beginning of menstruation. In Chinese medicine, this is explained as being due to the immaturity of the kidneys. Because the kidneys must supply essence to create the superabundance of blood necessary for menstruation to occur naturally, if the kidneys are not mature, they may not supply the needed essence every 28 days. Because maturation is not an all or nothing affair, as every parent knows, the amount of essence and, therefore, the regularity of the menstrual cycle may fluctuate for some time before it becomes stable. So it is said, "In adolescent (girls), blame the kidneys."

Once the kidneys have become stable and mature and menstruation occurs on a regular basis, then most gynecological diseases are impugned to the liver. In Chinese medicine, the liver is called the "temperamental viscus." This means that it is easily damaged or upset by emotional influences. In particular, it is said that, "The liver likes orderly reaching." This means that the liver qi likes to spread out without restriction or hindrance like a large broadleafed tree. When the liver encounters frustration, its coursing and discharging of the qi is inhibited. The qi cannot flow as freely as it wants and it becomes depressed and stagnant. The qi becomes bottled up, and this gives rise to anger and irritability since anger is the emotion associated with Chinese liver dis-ease.

42

However, when the qi becomes depressed and stuck, this also affects the flow of blood and body fluids, since it is the qi which moves and transforms both of these. Menstruation is the discharge of blood, and this discharge requires the free flow of qi to occur normally. Therefore, if the qi becomes depressed, the blood does not move, and if the blood does not move, menstruation cannot occur normally.

It is a fact of life that adults cannot do everything they want to do at the moment we want to do it. Learning to delay gratification is one of the things all adults learn, whether we like it or not. However, when we cannot do what we want to do when we want to do it, this affects our liver's coursing and discharging and the free spreading of our qi. Hence, it is a rare adult who has so few thwarted desires that their qi and blood flows absolutely freely and uninhibitedly. In actual clinical fact, almost all adults have some manifestations of liver depression qi stagnation, and in women, this almost always causes some menstrual irregularity. Therefore, because a certain level of liver depression qi stagnation is endemic in being an adult (at least in a civilized society where one must practice certain restraints), it is said, "In middle-aged (women), blame the liver."

According to the *Nei Jing (The Inner Classic)*, the "bible of Chinese medicine" compiled sometime in the second or third century BCE, the spleen and stomach begin to decline at around 35 years of age. Because the spleen and its helper the stomach are the source of the creation of qi and blood out of the food and liquids we eat, this decline in spleen-stomach function corresponds to a decline in the amounts of qi and blood produced. Therefore, from approximately 35 years of age till menopause, the spleen must struggle to produce enough qi and blood to nourish and empower the entire body and create a surplus of blood to flow over as the menstruate. This puts a heavy burden on the spleen and causes many women to show pronounced or more pronounced signs and symptoms of spleen weakness after the mid-30s and through the 40s. In such cases, the liver depression qi stagnation does not automatically go away. In fact, as we will see below, it may even get worse. However, when it comes to emphasis, this liver depression qi stagnation may not produce as many signs and symptoms as the spleen vacuity or weakness. Thus it is said, "In older (women), blame the spleen."[18]

As we will see in the next chapter, most breast diseases begin due to or at least involve liver depression qi stagnation. However, as a woman moves into her mid-30s and through her 40s, breast diseases are not just due to the liver but also due to the spleen and the other viscera and bowels associated with the spleen and liver, most notably the kidneys. Therefore, age plays its part in understanding the Chinese cause and treatment of breast disease and why breast diseases, such a premenstrual breast distention and pain, fibrocystic breasts, and even breast cancer, tend to occur more often and more severely in women as they age.

Menopause and Chinese medicine

Eventually, the body in its wisdom recognizes it is not healthy to try to create qi and blood to nourish and empower the rest of the body at the same time as continuing to menstruate regularly with the loss of blood that that necessarily entails. Therefore, the body initiates a transformation which, from the Chinese medical point of view, is literally a "change in life." The Chinese medical literature does not say exactly how, but at some point, the heart ceases sending blood down to collect in the uterus. Just as maturation does not happen all at once, this process is also a gradual one in most women. Therefore, the menses do not just suddenly cease, but menopause is commonly preceded by months

---

[18]   Obviously, 35 years of age or even 45 years of age is not considered old nowadays. The reader should keep in mind, however, that in ancient China when this saying was coined, due to hard physical labor, repeated and excessive pregnancies, and periodic famines and pestilences, many women were aged by their mid to late forties. In any case, these ages are not meant as absolutes but rather as a continuum, with spleen weakness becoming an important part of many women's Chinese medical diagnosis after approximately 35 years of age.

or even years of a certain amount of menstrual irregularity. Nevertheless, sooner or later, the heart stops sending blood down to the uterus. Instead, the kidneys are now free to send essence up to accumulate in the heart where it joins with the qi and blood sent up by the spleen and becomes spirit.

Thus the woman goes from mother of babies to mother of her tribe, the *sage femme* or wise woman full of spirit. If this change occurs smoothly, it naturally puts an end to any PMS and any breast conditions associated with PMS or which worsen during the premenstruum, since there is no menses let alone a pre-menses. Unfortunately, the smooth cessation of menstruation is, like all other transformations in the body, dependent on the free flow of liver qi. Since there is no PMS without liver depression qi stagnation[19], women's menopausal complaints tend to be, both in Chinese theory and my own clinical experience, proportional to the severity of their PMS. In other words, PMS, including premenstrual breast distention and pain and fibrocystic breasts, and menopausal syndrome are ultimately not two separate diseases but an unfortunate continuum whose core issue is liver depression qi stagnation. Readers interested in learning more about Chinese medicine and menopause should see my (Honora Lee Wolfe) *Menopause, A Second Spring: Making a Smooth Transition with Chinese Medicine* also published by Blue Poppy Press.

---

[19] Liver depression qi stagnation is the proper name of a pathological pattern in Chinese medicine. It is often abbreviated to either just liver depression or qi stagnation, or it may be referred to simply as liver qi. When speaking of the other four viscera or the bowels, if one says heart qi or spleen qi, one is referring to the healthy qi of that organ. But because the liver qi is so often depressed and stagnant in adults, this is the only case where simply saying liver qi almost always refers to a pathological condition of depression and stagnation.

PMS & Breast Disease

It should be obvious from the preceding discussion of Chinese medical physiology that the Chinese medical view of breast diseases is very different from that of Western medicine. According to Chinese medicine, *all the named Western diseases of the breast are considered to be due to the same or inter-related underlying disease mechanisms and are not really separate at all.* In other words, premenstrual breast pain and distention is only one stage of what may develop into other breast diseases such as breast lumps, whether painful or painless, or whether benign or malignant. This explains why some research suggests that women with what are considered by Western medicine to be benign breast diseases are more likely to develop breast cancer later in life. This progressive process is well delineated by Chinese medicine.

Chinese medical theory does *not suggest* that all women with one breast disorder *will* wind up with breast cancer. What Chinese medicine does say is that *breast diseases are related*, that most of them have similar disease mechanisms, that they can manifest as a continuum with varying routes, and that successful intervention can take place at most points along those routes *if a woman is willing to take responsibility for her own health.*

Chinese medicine sees premenstrual breast distention and pain as the starting point for most women's breast disease. Therefore, we need to understand the disease mechanisms of PMS if we are going to understand the disease mechanisms of breast disease.

The Chinese Mechanisms of PMS

The root cause of PMS is almost always a disharmony between the liver and spleen. Due to emotional stress and frustration, the liver becomes depressed and the qi becomes stagnant. Due to worry, lack of exercise, overfatigue, or improper diet, the spleen may become vacuous and weak. Because, in Chinese medicine, it is said that the liver controls the spleen, if the liver becomes depressed, this can cause or worsen spleen vacuity or weakness. Conversely, if the spleen is vacuous and weak, this may allow the liver to become or become even more depressed. Liver depression tends to worsen or arise during the premenstruum because the blood that was nourishing, softening, and harmonizing the liver is now being sent down to nourish the uterus. If there is not sufficient blood for both these purposes, the liver may not receive sufficient nourishment so that it can perform its duty of controlling the coursing and discharge, *i.e.*, the free flow, of the qi. If the liver does not course and discharge, the qi does not move freely and becomes stagnant.

If the qi does not flow freely, it backs up and accumulates. Like air filling a balloon, this accumulating qi has to go somewhere. If follows the liver channel and descends and accumulates in the lower abdomen, it causes premenstrual lower abdominal distention and pain. If it counterflows horizontally over the liver channel's network vessels in the chest, it causes premenstrual breast distention and pain and/or lateral costal distention and pain. And if it counterflows upward along the liver and gallbladder channels, it may give rise to premenstrual tension or migrainous headaches.

It is the spleen which is the root of qi and blood engenderment and transformation. If the spleen is vacuous and weak, then it may not engender and transform qi and blood sufficiently. If the spleen does not engender blood sufficiently, then, as we have just seen above, liver blood may become insufficient to allow the liver to perform its function of coursing and discharging the qi. On the other hand, if the spleen does not engender the qi sufficiently, the qi will lack its motivating force to move. Thus it is easy to see how closely these two viscera are related in terms of the free flow of the qi. The liver allows the qi to flow freely, but it is the spleen which is the ultimate source of the qi's power to move. Hence liver depression and spleen vacuity typically go hand in hand in clinical practice. In addition, we should remember that, because of their monthly loss of blood, women's spleens must work harder at producing blood then men's spleens must. This also predisposes women in particular towards a spleen insufficiency. In my experience (Bob Flaws), liver depression-spleen vacuity weakness is usually the root mechanism behind PMS. I have never seen a single case of PMS in 17 years of clinical practice without at least some element of liver depression.

According to Chinese medical theory, if the liver becomes depressed and qi stagnant, this may eventually transform into pathological heat. Remember that the qi is inherently warm. If the qi becomes stuck and accumulates, backing up under pressure, all this depressed and stagnant yang qi will transform into what is called transformative or depressive heat. Over time, this pathological heat, being by nature yang, will consume and dry out kidney yin. Since, in Chinese medicine, yin is supposed to control yang, if kidney yin becomes vacuous and weak, liver yang may become hyperactive. Since fire burns upward and the heart and lungs are located above the liver, this pathological heat may also accumulate in the heart, lungs, and/or breasts.

As mentioned above, since the spleen is the root of the engenderment and transformation of blood, if the spleen becomes weak, the blood may also become vacuous. Since some essence from the kidneys is required in order to make new blood, it is said in Chinese medicine that blood and essence share a common source. What this means in terms of disease mechanisms is that enduring blood vacuity may lead to insufficiency of kidney essence. This may aggravate any tendency to kidney yin vacuity already caused by damage due to enduring heat.

Because the spleen is also in charge of moving and transforming liquids, if the spleen becomes weak, water dampness may accumulate. Dampness which is yin, being thick and turbid, may further block the free flow of qi which is yang, thus aggravating liver depression. Dampness may also congeal and transform into phlegm. This phlegm even further impedes the free flow of qi and may lodge between the skin and flesh, in the channels and network vessels, and in what are known as the clear orifices of the heart and head. Phlegm blocking the clear orifices of the heart gives rise to mental emotional problems. Phlegm lodging in the breasts may give rise to hard, rubbery nodules there.

In Chinese medicine, the functioning of the spleen and stomach are likened to a pot on a stove and the process of digestion and the production of qi and blood is likened to the cooking of sour mash and distillation of alcohol. According to this metaphor, qi and blood are the distillation of foods and liquids cooked and transformed by the spleen and stomach. However, the ultimate source of heat for the spleen and stomach to do their job is the kidney fire or kidney yang. This kidney fire can be likened to the pilot light in a stove. If it goes out, the burners cannot function. Therefore, if the spleen remains chronically weak, since kidney yang is the source of the heat of the middle burner, *i.e.*, the spleen and stomach, kidney yang may also become weak. Since kidney essence is the material basis of both kidney yin and yang, this process can be accelerated if there is long-term blood vacuity. On the other hand, enduring kidney yang vacuity and weakness will also impair blood production as well.

Even if one cannot grasp the meanings and implications of all of the above on their first reading, the reader should by now agree that Chinese medicine is by no means a primitive folk medicine. There are even a few more mechanisms at work in some women's PMS which may occur as ramifications of these main disease mechanisms. However, the above mechanisms are the root of most premenstrual signs and symptoms, including all premenstrual breast disease or breast disease whose symptoms worsen during the premenstruum. If one understands these mechanisms and has a sound grasp of the basic theories of Chinese medicine discussed above, one can figure out *a rational explanation for any sign or symptom any woman may experience before her menses.* For more information on PMS in general, interested readers may see my (Bob Flaws's) *Curing PMS Naturally with Chinese Medicine.*

The six depressions & breast disease

There is one last Chinese medical theory we need to have some familiarity with before we can fully understand the Chinese medical mechanisms of all breast diseases. This is Zhu Dan-xi's theory of the six depressions which we actually have already touched upon. According to this famous Yuan dynasty Chinese medical thinker, six main things can become depressed or get stuck in the body. These are the qi, blood, dampness, phlegm, food, and fire. In addition, stagnations of these six things in the body are not isolated events but tend to be interrelated.

Qi stagnation

We have already seen that if, due to emotional stress, the liver loses its coursing and discharge, the qi may become stagnant and back up. We have also seen how such a qi stagnation may cause breast distention and pain in the breasts because of channels and network vessels connecting the liver with the breasts.

Blood stasis

The blood may become depressed or static due to any of a number of causes. Trauma may damage the vessels allowing the blood to seep outside them. Since the blood can only flow as long as it stays in the channels and network vessels according to Chinese medicine, this extravasated blood becomes static. However, the blood can also become static for a number of other reasons as well. There may be insufficient qi to propel the blood. There may be insufficient blood to nourish the vessels and keep them

51

properly working. Or there may be qi stagnation. As mentioned above:

> The qi moves the blood. If the qi moves, the blood moves. If the qi stops, the blood stops.

Therefore, long-term or serious qi stagnation can give rise to blood stasis. Blood stasis may also be caused or aggravated by dampness, phlegm, or food. Any of these other three material substances may block and hinder the flow of qi and, therefore, the free and uninhibited flow of blood.

Damp obstruction

If body fluids do not flow freely and accumulate, they may transform from healthy, moistening fluids to pathological dampness. Such dampness may be due to external invasion from the outside, for stance, due to living in a damp environment, or may be engendered internally due to eating too many "damp" foods, such as sugar and fat, and too little exercise. Once dampness has been engendered, being a yin substance, it tends to obstruct the free flow of yang qi. Therefore, dampness can cause or aggravate qi stagnation.

Phlegm congelation

If dampness becomes depressed and stagnates and this endures, it may congeal into phlegm. Since phlegm is even a more dense material than dampness, I tends to obstruct the free flow of qi and, therefore, blood and healthy body fluids, even more strongly than simple dampness.

Food stagnation

It is qi's job to move and transform food. If one overeats or eats too many hard-to-digest foods, such as meat, cheese, and nuts, the food may not be dispersed and transformed but rather stagnate and accumulate. Like blood, dampness, and phlegm, yin food may block the flow of yang qi and, consequently give rise to or aggravate qi stagnation or aggravate the preceding three yin depressions.

Depressive fire

We have already seen when discussing PMS that qi stagnation may, if it endures long enough or is severe enough, transform into evil heat or fire. Heat's nature is yang and tends to travel upward. Therefore, depressive heat or fire tends to affect the organs and tissues in the upper part of the body, including the breasts.

As we have seen above, it is qi's job to transport and transform the blood, body fluids, phlegm, and food. Therefore, qi stagnation may cause or aggravate blood stasis, damp obstruction, phlegm congelation, or food stagnation. Conversely, any of these four may block and obstruct the free flow of qi. Thus it is common to see qi stagnation *and* blood stasis, damp obstruction *and* qi stagnation, phlegm congelation *and* qi stagnation, and qi *and* food stagnation. However, if one has qi stagnation, then it is also easy to develop depressive heat or fire. In that case, one may get depressive heat and blood stasis, damp heat, phlegm, heat, and food stagnation plus depressive heat.

Basically, the overwhelming majority of breast diseases are nothing other than varying proportions of these six depressions or stagnations occurring in the breasts. If there is just swelling and distention, there may only be qi stagnation and dampness. If there is pain, there is heat and/or stasis. If there are lumps, there is blood stasis and/or phlegm nodulation. And in some cases, at least five out of six depressions exist simultaneously.

Treatment According to Pattern Discrimination

The hallmark of professional Chinese medicine is what is known as "treatment based on pattern discrimination." Modern Western medicine bases its treatment on a disease diagnosis. This means that two patients diagnosed as suffering from the same disease will get the same treatment. Traditional Chinese medicine also takes the patient's disease diagnosis into account. However, the choice of treatment is not based on the disease so much as it is on what is called the patient's pattern, and it is treatment based on pattern discrimination which is what makes Chinese medicine the holistic, safe, and effective medicine it is.

In order to explain the difference between a disease and pattern, let us take headache for example. Everyone who is diagnosed as suffering from a headache has to, by definition, have some pain in their head. In modern Western medicine and other medical systems which primarily prescribe on the basis of a disease diagnosis, one can talk about "headache medicines." However, amongst headache sufferers, one may be a man and the other a woman. One may be old and the other young. One may be fat and the other skinny. One may have pain on the right side of her head and the other may have pain on the left. In one case, the pain may be throbbing and continuous, while the other person's pain may be very sharp but intermittent. In one case, they may also have indigestion, a tendency to loose stools, lack of warmth in their feet, red eyes, a dry mouth and desire for cold drink, while the other person has a wet, weeping, crusty skin rash with red borders, a tendency to hay fever, ringing in their ears, and dizziness when they stand up. In Chinese medicine just as in modern Western medicine, both these patients suffer from headache. That is their disease diagnosis. However, they also suffer from a whole host of other complaints, have very different types of headaches, and very different constitutions, ages, and sex. In Chinese medicine, the patient's pattern is made up from all these other signs and symptoms and other information. Thus, in Chinese medicine, the pattern describes *the totality of the person as a unique individual.* And in Chinese medicine, treatment is designed to rebalance that entire pattern of imbalance as well as address the major complaint or disease. Thus, there is a saying in Chinese medicine:

One disease, different treatments
Different diseases, same treatment

This means that, in Chinese medicine, two patients with the same named disease diagnosis may receive different treatments *if their Chinese medical patterns are different,* while two patients diagnosed with different named diseases may receive the same treatment *if their Chinese medical pattern is the same.* In other words, in Chinese medicine, treatment is predicated primarily on one's pattern discrimination, not on one's named disease diagnosis. Therefore, each person is treated individually. In professionally practiced Chinese medicine, there is no one fibroadenoma or breast cancer formula or herb. Nor is there is any one magic breast disease acupuncture point. Each patient's Chinese herbal or acupuncture formula is individually crafted for their particular pattern with their particular disease being of secondary importance.

Since every patient gets just the treatment which is right to restore balance to their particular body, there are also no unwanted side effects. Side effects come from forcing one part of the body to behave while causing an imbalance in some other part. The medicine may have fit part of the problem but not the entirety of the patient as an individual. This is like robbing Peter to pay Paul. Since Chinese medicine sees the entire body (and mind!) as a single, unified whole, curing imbalance in one area of the body while causing it in another is unacceptable.

Below is a description of the major Chinese medical patterns at work in the benign breast diseases. These are first given as pure patterns in their textbook form. Then we will go on to give a more real-life account of what is seen in clinical practice. If you suffer from breast disease, you will probably recognize a number of your symptoms under one or more of the patterns below. Note that the treatment principles under each pattern are different. No single treatment will work for every woman with breast disease.

1. Liver depression, qi stagnation

This pattern forms the basis of all the other patterns of breast pain and distention (*ru fang zhang tong*) and mammary aggregation (*ru pi*), the traditional Chinese term for fibrocystic breasts. As a pure pattern, it is mostly seen in younger women or in the first stages of the breast disease.

Signs and symptoms: Emotional depression, lack of fulfillment of one's heart's desires, irritability, breast distention and pain, chest and lateral costal distention and pain, frequent sighing, menstrual irregularity, possible lower abdominal distention and pain at the onset of menstruation, a normal colored tongue with thin, white (*i.e.*, normal fur), and bowstring pulse

Disease mechanisms: "The liver is the temperamental viscus." If one experiences unrelieved stress or frustration, liver qi will be unable to flow smoothly and the subjective experience of this is depression and irritability. If the qi flow is not smooth or if the qi is trapped in the upper body, it may affect the breasts, flanks, and ribs or upper back. The frequent sighing is the attempt of the woman to relieve this pent up qi. The harmonious or smooth and even coursing and discharge of the liver qi controls the liver storage of the blood and hence the timing and regularity of the menstruation. Therefore, if the liver qi loses its harmony, the menstrual cycle may become irregular. It is said in Chinese medicine:

> If there is free flow, there is no pain. If there is pain, there is no free flow.

In this case, dysmenorrhea at the onset of menstruation is due to the lack of free flow of the qi in turn due to liver depression qi stagnation. The liver channel runs through the uterus and lower abdomen, and dysmenorrhea is a very common symptom of liver depression in women. Likewise, the bowstring or wiry pulse shows that there is lack of relaxed, free flow, while a slightly dark tongue also shows the same thing.

Treatment principles: Course the liver and rectify the qi

2. Liver-stomach depressive heat

Signs and symptoms: All the same signs and symptoms of the above pattern *plus* more breast pain and inflammation, possible inflamed or painful nipples, easy anger and not just irritability, a bitter taste in the mouth, increased hunger, possible premenstrual acne, possible easy crying, a bitter taste in the morning, a dark red tongue with yellow fur, and a rapid, bowstring pulse

Disease mechanisms: The liver and stomach share a number of close relationships as do their respective channels. If liver depression endures and transforms into heat, this may counterflow horizontally to invade the stomach. This then causes a loss of the stomach's harmony and upward counterflow of both the liver and stomach qi. The stomach channel traverses the breasts and an internal channel of the liver goes to the nipples. Therefore, there is pain and inflammation of these tissues, not simply distention. This depressive heat manifests as red pimples on the chin and around the mouth, the course of the stomach channel. Likewise, the increased hunger suggests heat in the stomach. The easy crying is due to this heat also disturbing the function of the lungs, while the bitter taste in the mouth, the red tongue

58

with yellow coating and the rapidity of the pulse all po: existence of pathological heat.

Treatment principles: Course the liver and harmonize the stomach, clear heat and resolve depression

This is a commonly seen pattern in younger women with a reasonably robust physique.

3. Liver depression with spleen vacuity

Signs and symptoms: All the same signs and symptoms listed in #1 plus fatigue, loose stools, reduced appetite or a craving for sweets, nausea, abdominal distention after meals, cold hands and feet, possible edematous swelling, a fat tongue with teeth prints along its edges, and a wiry, fine pulse

Disease mechanisms: If the liver becomes depressed, it may counterflow horizontally to assail the spleen as well as the stomach. Whereas the stomach typically becomes hot and replete, the spleen becomes vacuous and weak. This is evidenced by the fatigue, loose stools, nausea, abdominal distention after meals, cold hands and feet, the edematous swelling, and the fat tongue. These last two signs show that the spleen is too weak to control the movement and transformation of body fluids. The fine pulse is due to blood vacuity in turn due to spleen vacuity.

Treatment principles: Course the liver and rectify the qi, fortify the spleen and boost the qi

This pattern becomes very common as women reach their mid to late 30's. However, in real-life it is not uncommon to see a combination of liver-stomach depressive heat plus spleen vacuity.

4. Liver depression with liver blood-kidney yin vacuity

Signs and symptoms: There is premenstrual breast distention, chest oppression, low back and knee soreness and weakness, possible late menarche (over 16 yrs.), a thin physique, dizziness, tinnitus, night sweats, heat in the palms of the hands and soles of the feet, vexation and agitation, insomnia or dream-disturbed sleep, early and/or scanty menstruation, a pale red tongue with red tongue tip and scanty, possibly yellow, dry fur, and a fine, rapid, bowstring pulse.

Disease mechanisms: These signs and symptoms are a mixture of liver depression qi stagnation signs and symptoms and liver blood-kidney yin vacuity symptoms. Because yin controls yang, if yin becomes vacuous and insufficient, if may fail to control yang. Yang then flushes upward and outward, thus giving rise to the heat in the hands and feet, night sweats, vexation and agitation, dream-disturbed sleep, tinnitus, and dizziness. The tongue is pale because of the blood vacuity, while its tip is red and the fur is yellow and dry because of the heat rising upward in the body. The pulse is fine due to blood and yin vacuity, rapid due to yin failing to control yang, and bowstring due to the liver depression.

Treatment principles: Enrich the kidneys and nourish the liver, course the liver and rectify the qi

That being said, although one can comes across this pattern in its pure form, it commonly presents combined with spleen qi and often even kidney yang vacuity as well. When seen in its pure form, it is mostly in very thin, very anxious and high-strung young women.

6. Liver depression with liver blood & kidney yang vacuity

Signs and symptoms: Breast distention, lower back and knee soreness and weakness, fatigue, low or no sex drive, cold feet, frequent urination or night-time urination, a pale tongue with white coating, and a bowstring, fine, slow, and/or deep pulse

Disease mechanism: The breast distention and bowstring pulse are due to liver depression qi stagnation, while the other symptoms are all reflective of the kidney yang vacuity. The warmth of the lower body and the strength of the sex drive are very much rooted the kidney yang.

Treatment principles: Nourish the liver and invigorate the kidneys, warm yang and rectify the qi

Although all textbooks include this pattern, it is never really seen in this form in Western women. Most women's spleen and kidneys (both yin and yang) get weak and insufficient in their 40's and early 50's. The liver depression and even either yin vacuity/vacuity heat or depressive heat may also be present. Therefore, one does not usually see the pale tongue or the deep, slow pulse.

7. Blood stasis

As we have seen above, long-term qi stagnation may lead to blood stasis, while long-term qi stagnation and spleen vacuity may lead to damp accumulation and phlegm congelation or nodulation. If blood stasis complicates any of the above patterns, there are hard lumps with well-defined borders. They may or may not be painful. The tongue will usually become dark and possibly purplish. Often there will be other signs of blood stasis, like varicose veins, red dots on the skin (tiny hemangiomas), brown spots on the face and hands, etc.

Treatment principles: Quicken the blood and dispel stasis

8. Phlegm nodulation

If there is phlegm nodulation, there will be cystic lumps which tend to be well-defined, movable, and painful or not painful. The pulse will be slippery among its other qualities, and the person will typically have a history of excessive phlegm production, for example allergies, sinusitis, or asthma.

Treatment principles: Transform phlegm, soften the hard, and scatter nodulation

9. Heat toxins

If depressive becomes more virulent, it may transform into toxic heat. The symptoms of toxic heat include localized swelling, pain, and redness, pus or purulence, and open sores or ulcers. We will talk more about toxins when we discuss cancer *per se.*

Treatment principles: Clear heat and resolve toxins

For women in their 40's with liver depression and spleen-kidney dual vacuity with an element of heat, phlegm nodulation, and blood stasis, a more typical description of signs and symptoms would include: premenstrual breast distention which has gotten worse with age, fibrocystic lumps which get larger and sore as menstruation approaches, premenstrual irritability *and* tearfulness, acne, fatigue, loose stools, possible weight gain, premenstrual low back pain, cold feet, decreased sex drive, nighttime urination, possible insomnia and/or heart palpitations, occasional hot flashes, early menstruation which is scanty in amount, period pain, the expulsion of dark clots in the menstruate, a dark, fat tongue with teeth marks on its edges and scanty, slightly yellow fur, and a wiry, fine pulse which is slippery and floating in its most distal positions.

Treatment principles: Course the liver and resolve depression, nourish the liver and invigorate the kidneys, quicken the blood and dispel stasis, transform phlegm and scatter nodulation, clear whatever kind or amount of heat is present from wherever in the body

Why breast diseases tend to worsen with age

There is a saying in Chinese medicine that new breast diseases or those in younger women are due to the liver, while enduring breast diseases or those in older women are due to the *chong mai*. The *chong mai* is one of the so-called eight extraordinary vessels, and menstruation is intimately connected with the proper functioning of this vessel. When this vessel becomes exuberant at puberty, menstruation commences, and when it becomes exhausted at the climacteric, the menstruation pauses. This vessel connects the kidneys and uterus with the heart, chest, and upper body. The *chong mai* carries blood from the heart down to the uterus and yin essence upward from the kidneys to become heart spirit above. In terms of menstruation, the *chong mai* functions properly when the heart, spleen, liver, and kidneys function properly.

Therefore, saying that enduring breast diseases or breast diseases in older women have to do with the *chong mai* is only a way of saying that in those cases, there is more than just liver depression qi stagnation going on. In those cases, the liver, spleen, and kidneys are all affected. As we have seen above, the spleen and kidneys frequently become weak and insufficient in women beginning in their mid-30s and worsening in their 40's and early 50's. Because of this liver depression also tends to get worse. Therefore, breast diseases also tend to get worse during this same time frame. This explains both the worsening of PMS, the worsening of fibrocystic breasts, and the increased incidence of breast cancer.

I (Bob Flaws) have treated hundreds of Western women in their late 30's, 40's, and early 50's. In such cases, the single most common Chinese medical pattern I see is a combination of liver depression and spleen and kidney vacuity complicated by varying amounts of heat, blood stasis, damp obstruction, and phlegm nodulation. Although different patients have different proportions of these, many patients do have elements of all these

63

together. In that case, one must treat the entire pattern in order to get the right result. Treating only the liver depression, spleen vacuity, the kidney vacuity, the blood stasis, or the phlegm nodulation does not get a satisfactory result.

This means that Chinese medicine agrees with those Western clinicians who now say that fibrocystic breast condition and breast cancer are conditions associated with aging. Unlike Western medicine, Chinese medicine stills considers fibrocystic breasts a disease and does offer safe and effective treatments for it. In addition, these same treatments are believed to have some effect for preventing the development of breast cancer.

The Chinese Medical View
of Breast Cancer

In premodern times, breast cancer was called *ru yan* or breast rock in Chinese.[20] This is because it was undiagnosable in ancient times until a rock-hard, tortoise-shell like tumor was palpable. Although there is no distinction in traditional Chinese medicine between benign and malignant diseases the same way there is in modern Western medicine, breast rock was known to be an incurable disease.

The *locus classicus* or classical discussion of breast cancer is found in the work of the same Yuan dynasty doctor who first discussed the six depression above, Zhu Dan-xi. In speaking of breast rock, Zhu said:

> If (a woman) is out of favor with her husband, her brother, or her sister-in-law, worry and anger, depression and oppression will accumulate day and night. The spleen qi will be dispersed and impeded and the liver qi will counterflow wildly. As a result, a dormant node will develop gradually as big as a chess piece with no pain or itching.

> It takes tens of years to develop into a sudden sore, called suckling breast rock because it forms a depression like a rock cave. (This) is then incurable. If, *at the initial stage of its generation*, (one) eliminates the root of the disease by keeping the heart tranquil and the spirit calm and then carries out a (proper)

---

[20] Jia Kun, *Carcinoma*, The Commercial Press, Hong Kong, 1985, p. 98

treatment method, there is the possibility of healing.[21] [Parentheses ours]

The above passages are pregnant with meaning. First of all, Zhu is saying that the main cause of breast cancer is emotional stress and frustration. Secondly, he says that the disease mechanism primarily involves the spleen and liver. Third, he says that it takes tens of years for this disease to manifest. And fourth, and perhaps most importantly, Zhu says that, if one eliminates the root cause (*i.e.*, emotional stress and frustration), keeps one spirit calm, and gives proper treatment, this disease mechanism may be cured or aborted before it gets to the stage of incurable breast rock.

This basic theory about the cause and mechanisms of breast cancer has continued down through the centuries to be the core belief in Chinese medicine. In the *Wai Ke Zheng Zhi (The Orthodox Manual of External Disease)* of the Ming dynasty (1368-1644 CE), it is pointed out that:

> Breast cancer is due to worry and melancholy. Lots of ideas hanging around make one feel dissatisfied. Perverse flow of liver *qi* to the spleen leads to the obstruction of the channels....[22]

Even the contemporary Chinese textbook on the treatment of cancer, *Carcinoma* by Jia Kun, reiterates this fact:

> Breast cancer is mainly caused by the disturbed emotions such as grief, bitter weeping, fear, worry and depression, or by improper sexual life without paying attention to hygiene, or by increased excretion of estrogen. It is also closely related to artificial abortion, early terminated pregnancy, single life, no breast feeding and improper breast feeding. After menopause, the

---

[21] *Extra Treatises Based on Inquiry & Investigation.*, by Zhu Dan-xi, trans. By Yang Shou-zhong, Blue Poppy Press, May, 1994, p. 63-64

[22] Zhang, Dai-zhao, *The Treatment of Cancer By Integrated Chinese-Western Medicine*, Blue Poppy Press, Boulder, CO, 1989, p. 18

deteriorated function of the nervous system, the impaired excretion of ovarian hormone, the blocked regulation of the ovaries by nervous system and some other diseases can also result in breast cancer.[23]

Jia Kun "mixes his metaphors" in the passage above, combining both Chinese and Western disease mechanisms of this disease. However, when it comes to the Chinese disease mechanisms, the emphasis is on the woman's emotional health. Emotional frustration, depression, suppressed anger, and stress affect the free and uninhibited flow of the liver qi. The liver becomes depressed and the qi becomes stagnant. Because of the connection between the liver and stomach channels and the liver channel and the nipples as well as the connection between the liver and the *chong mai* and the *chong mai* and the breasts, liver depression qi stagnation may result in qi stagnation in the breasts. Because the qi moves the blood and body fluids, either or both of these may accumulate and become stagnant in the breasts. If the blood stops moving in the breasts, it results in blood stasis, while if the body fluids stop moving in the breasts, they may congeal into phlegm. In either case, these yin depressions further hinder the free flow of yang qi and may give rise to the local arising of depressive heat. This is nothing other than the same mechanisms of benign breast disease we have talked about above.

The Difference Between Benign & Malignant Breast Disease

If the basic disease mechanisms between benign and malignant breast diseases are essentially the same, why do some women only develop benign fibrocystic breasts while other develop progressive, terminal cancer? It is extremely important that we

---

[23] Jia Kun, *op. cit.*, p. 98

answer this question. Only if we do can we then go on to create rationale regimes to prevent breast cancer.

Dr. Sun Bing-yan is one of the most famous traditional Chinese doctors specializing in cancer alive today. According to Dr. Sun, there is no cancer unless there are "toxins." The concept of toxins is an ancient one. In Chinese medicine, toxins are especially virulent disease evils. In most cases, they are hot in nature. Frequently, they are both damp and hot. They often reside or hide in the blood. When they become active, they corrode or destroy the body's healthy qi, blood, body fluids, and tissues, causing ulcers, necrotic (or dead) tissue, pus and purulence. Dr. Sun quotes Hua Tuo, the most famous Chinese doctor of the Han dynasty (circa 200 CE) when he says that,

> a tumor is not only caused by the stagnation of Qi and blood, but also by the accumulated toxin in the five Zang (*i.e.*, viscera) and six Fu (bowels). This viewpoint distinguished the tumor from the common stagnation of Qi, blood, phlegm, and indigestion (*i.e.*, food stagnation)... What this means is that if there is only Qi, blood, phlegm and indigestion but without cancer toxin, there will be no tumor disease.[24] [Parentheses ours]

Dr. Sun then goes on to quote the Song dynasty (960-1280 CE) Chinese doctor, Yang Shi-ying, who reiterates this idea:

> Cancer may sink like a cave or bump up like a mountain. The root of the toxin is so deep and hidden that it can spread out in various directions of the body.[25]

Where do these toxins come from? In all probability, environmental and chemical pollutants play a part in the creation of cancer toxins in the body. Because Chinese medical theory was mostly

---

[24] Sun, Bingyan, *Cancer Treatment and Prevention (with Traditional Chinese Medicine)*, Offete Enterprises, Inc., San Mateo, CA, 1991, p. 6

[25] *Ibid.*, p. 6

created before the Industrial Revolution, the concept of environmental toxins is not well developed within it. However, Chinese did know that lacquer workers often became diseased due to "lacquer toxins." Therefore, there is room within Chinese medical theory to develop the concept of chemical and environmental toxins more fully in the future. If environmental pollutants and chemical contamination play a role in the cause of breast cancer, as they most probably do, then minimizing exposure to such chemicals and pollutants is the obvious preventive step.

But Sun Bing-yan says that these cancer toxins are also internally generated. As we have seen above, if the qi becomes blocked, it may back up behind this blockage. Because qi is inherently warm, if such stagnation becomes severe enough or endures long enough, it may transform from simple qi stagnation to depressive heat. If, due the interrelationship between the qi and body fluids, this depressive heat becomes involved with pathological dampness, damp heat may be engendered. If this damp heat becomes associated with blood stasis and the body's righteous or healthy qi is so weak that it cannot combat it successfully, this damp heat may further "implode", becoming heat or damp heat toxins.

According to Dr. Sun, such transformation of qi stagnation into heat or damp heat toxins is inversely proportional to the health of the spleen. This is because, as we have seen above, one of the spleen's main roles is for its qi to move and transform body fluids. If, due to any reason, the spleen qi becomes vacuous and weak, the spleen may fail in its function of moving and transporting fluids and humors. These then may collect and transform into pathological or so-called evil dampness which then obstructs the free flow of liver qi.

We have also seen above that the free flow of liver qi is also dependent on the propelling power of the spleen qi. In addition, the function of the liver is likewise dependent on the warming function of the kidneys. Kidney yang, also called the life gate fire, provides the warmth which allows the liver to function, remem-

69

bering that all physiological functions in the body are warm transformations according to Chinese medicine. Although it may seem contradictory that a decrease in the yang qi of the spleen and kidneys may make the transformation of depressive heat and, therefore, heat toxins more likely, this is an ancient and well-accepted theory in Chinese medicine called Li Dong-yuan's theory of yin fire.

What this means is that those women who have more liver depression and qi stagnation *plus* more spleen qi and kidney yang vacuity are more likely to engender yin fire. If this yin fire is severe enough, it may create heat toxins, and, according to Dr. Sun, it is the presence of heat toxins which distinguishes breast cancer from other, benign breast diseases.

The Implications of This Theory

In terms of prevention, there are a number of important implications of the above theory on the Chinese cause and mechanisms of breast cancer. First, anything which promotes free flow of the liver qi systemically is going to be beneficial. This can be done by "keeping the spirit calm" in the frst place but also by proper exercise and diet as well as other professionally supplied treatments, such as acupuncture and Chinese herbal medicine. Secondly, anything which keeps the qi and, therefore, the blood and body fluids flowing normally to and through the breasts is going to be beneficial, and there are a number of both professionally applied and self-care treatments which can do just that. And third, anything which keeps the spleen and kidneys healthy is also going to be very important. Exercise, diet, and Chinese herbal medicine can all promote the health of the spleen, while Chinese herbs and moxibustion are useful for keeping the kidneys strong and healthy. Conversely, anything which either depresses the liver, weakens the spleen, or exhausts the kidneys should be avoided or minimized. Knowing this, we now can formulate a plan of action.

9

The Three Free Therapies

Introduction

Breast disease can be treated and, more importantly, it can be prevented. There are Chinese medical treatment plans for all the above-mentioned patterns associated with breast disease. Remedially, these treatments typically involve Chinese herbs or acupuncture therapy which must be administered professionally. However, in the Tang dynasty (circa 700 CE), there was a famous Chinese physician named Sun Si-miao who said that a physician should first and foremost be an educator of society. He believed that initial treatment should involve adjustment of the patient's diet and lifestyle. Only if that failed to affect a cure should other treatment be given.

Therefore, in our clinic, we stress what we have come to call "The Three Free Therapies." These are deep relaxation, exercise, and proper diet. They are free because only you can do them for yourself. These three free therapies can help in keeping any woman free from PMS and menstrual diseases in general and breast diseases in particular. They are based on a combination of Chinese medical theory and simple common sense and can form the basis of *anyone's* health regime or lifestyle. They can (and probably should) be practiced throughout one's life, free of charge.

Deep Relaxation

The single most important part of any treatment program for keeping the qi and blood in the whole body free-flowing is daily

relaxation. This therapy, if done consistently and with perseverance, can make a difference not only in terms of symptoms but
one's fundamental character and *modus operandi* in the world.
The reason this therapy is so effective is that it addresses *at the
root* the effects of stress and emotional upsetment which are
involved in all problems with a component of liver depression qi
stagnation. In most cases having such an emotional component,
I (Honora Lee Wolfe) believe this therapy can be as or even more
beneficial than a good deal of currently available psychotherapy.

Please do not misunderstand. I (Honora Lee Wolfe) have personally experienced useful psychotherapeutic work, and sometimes
may recommend both psychotherapy *and* daily relaxation to a
client. However, many forms of "talk" therapy allow or even
foster the patient going over and over and over their problems,
both real and fabricated, in such as way as to foster the continua-
tion of the same types of thought patterns over and over and over
again. This does not eradicate the problem, nor does it often deal
with the person's real problems at all. I am not anti-psychother-
apy in all cases, but I also believe that whatever happened that
makes one frustrated or angry is better released in one moment
and forgotten in the next.

One can do little about the traffic, one's mother's manipulative
behavior when one was a child, or the fact that the boss was in a
bad mood this morning. However, it is better to let go of the
emotions associated with these events as much as possible and
do what needs to be done in one's life. That may include moving
away from where your mother lives or changing jobs. Holding
onto the anger and frustration is not useful and, hopefully, we
have demonstrated that it is deleterious to your health. Regular
daily programmed deep relaxation can help anyone learn how to
let go. Once one lets go, the qi will automatically flow freely and
in the proper directions.

In our culture stress is endemic—job stress, political stress,
environmental pollution stress, relationship stress, sexual stress,
nuclear warfare stress, the stress of the constant decisions

required by living in a "free" society. We have created a society which produces more stress than the human body can process and still remain healthy. Past a certain age, most of us will develop at least some symptoms due to this fact. These symptoms may come and go and we can learn to keep them largely under control, but it is arrogant and unreasonable to think that we can forever keep up the often frenetic pace (physically or emotionally) which many of us must in order to survive and still be free of the ravages of stress.

Women especially find themselves at a time and place in history with "unlimited" options, where our roles are multiple and our sense of self often ill-defined. Our family structure is weaker and less supportive than at any time in American history; community support for parenting is inadequate; divorce is endemic; and the stay-at-home mother-and-housewife is no longer an option in most cases. The sexual confusion wrought by the '60s and '70s is even worse with the arrival of life-threatening sexually transmitted diseases. The constant demands on the time of the average 35-50 year old woman in our society often leaves us with no "down" time and the feeling of being always behind, always pushed, always squeezed.

Daily deep relaxation therapy is one way to turn off the heat under the boiler of stress, to loosen the grip of the vise producing that squeezed feeling, and to lessen the toll that these pressures take on our health.

Based on research done at sanatoria and hospitals in China, in order for deep relaxation therapy to have measurable clinical effectiveness there are a few criteria which must be met.

1. It must result in somatic, physical relaxation as well as mental relaxation.

2. It must result in the center of consciousness coming out of one's head and into some part of the lower body, preferably the area of the lower abdomen.

73

3. It must be done a minimum of 20 minutes at a single stretch per day, although no longer than 30 minutes are required.

4. It must be done every day without missing a single day for *at least* 100 days.

There are many possible techniques which will accomplish this type of deep relaxation, including hatha yoga, meditation, and biofeedback. The easiest way, however, is to purchase one or two relaxation or stress reduction tapes available at health food stores and "new age" bookstores. These take about 25-30 minutes each, are relatively inexpensive, and require minimal discipline.

Some people say that they cannot relax, that it is very difficult for them to keep their mind concentrated during meditation, or that they do not have time to relax. It is precisely these people who need to relax the most. These tapes are helpful for these people, in that, to some extent, they supply the needed concentration. Each time the mind wanders, the tape brings one back to the task at hand so that one does not need to concentrate on anything. All one has to do is to listen to the tape.

Additionally, it is best to try to do the tape at the same time each day, so that, after a while it becomes like eating, getting dressed, or brushing your teeth—in other words, a nondiscretionary part of your day.

At the end of three months, if you have done such deep relaxation every day without missing a day, you may expect to be calmer and less flappable. In addition, based on Chinese research, your appetite should be better, your energy should be beeter, your sleep should be better, the temperature in your hands and feet shouyld be more normal, and your blood pressure should be more normal. These are not inconsequential changes for the better in anyone's health![26] At the end of three years of regular practice (*i.e.*, 1,000 days), one will be a different person altogether.

Regular Exercise

For exercise to be most effective for liver depression qi stagnation, it is better if it is aerobic in nature. That means it must increase your heart rate 80% above your resting rate and keep it there for at least 20 minutes. Like the deep relaxation, no further health gains are made after 30 minutes. To calculate your normal resting heart rate, place your fingers over the pulsing artery on the front side of your neck. Count the beats for 15 seconds and then multiply by four. This gives you your beats per minute or BPM. Now multiply your BPM by 0.8. Take the resulting number and add it to your resting BPM. This gives you your aerobic threshold of BPM. Next engage in any physical activity you like.

After you have been exercising for five minutes, take your pulse for 15 seconds once again at the artery on the front side of your throat. Again multiply the resulting count by four and this tells you your current BPM. If this number is less than your aerobic threshold BPM, then you know you need to exercise harder or faster. Once you get your heart rate up to your aerobic threshold, then you need to keep exercising at the same level of intensity for at least 20 minutes. In order to insure that one is keeping their heartbeat high enough for long enough, one should recount their pulse every five minutes or so.

Depending on one's age and physical condition, different women will have to exercise harder to reach their aerobic threshold than others. For some women, simply walking briskly will raise their heartbeat 80% above their resting rate. For other women, they will need to do calisthenics, running, swimming, racquetball, or

---

[26] Benson, Herbert, *The Relaxation Response*, G.K. Hall & Co., Boston, 1976, p. 86-87

some other, more strenuous exercise. It really does not matter what the exercise is as long as it raises your heartbeat 80% above your resting rate and keeps it there for 20 minutes. However, there are two other criteria that should be met. One, the exercise should be something that is not too boring. If it is too boring, you may have a hard time keeping up your schedule. Since most people do find aerobic exercises such as running, stationary bicycles, and stair-steppers boring, it is good to listen to music or watch TV in order to distract your mind from the tedium.

Secondly, the type of exercise should not cause any damage to any parts of the body. For instance, running on pavement may cause knee problems for some people. Therefore, you should pick a type of exercise you enjoy but also one which will not cause any problems.

When doing aerobic exercise, it is best to exercise either every day or every other day. Doing aerobics only once every 72 hours will have minimal cumulative effects. Therefore, we recommend women with breast disease to do some sort of aerobic exercises every day or every other day, three to four times per week *at least*. The good news is that there is no real need to exercise more than 30 minutes at any one time. Forty-five minutes per session is not going to be all that much better than 25 minutes per session. And 25 minutes four times per week is much better than one hour once a week.

Recent research has also demonstrated that weight-lifting can help relieve emotional depression in women of all ages.[27] Therefore, we have begun recommending lifting weights on the days when one is not doing aerobics. In that case, one can do aerobics three to four days a week and lift weights the other three days. In general, one should not lift weights every day unless one

---

[27] "Depression and Weight Training", *Harvard Women's Health Watch*, Vol. IV, #6, February 1997, reporting on research published in the *Journal of Gerontology*, January 1997

varies the muscle groups they are working each day. In the study on weight-lifting and depression cited above, the women lifted weights which were 45-87% as heavy as the maximum they could lift at one time. Those women who lifted weights closer to the top end of this range saw the greatest benefits. These women lifted weights three days per week for 10 weeks, gradually increasing the amount of weight they lifted at each session.

Because weight-lifting requires some initial training and education in order to do it safely and properly, we recommend taking a few classes either at a local YMCA or recreation center or from a private trainer. When aerobics are alternated with weight-lifting, one has a really comprehensive training regime designed to benefit both one's cardiovascular system and one's muscles, tendons, ligaments, and bones. In addition, regular weight-bearing exercise is also important for preventing osteoporosis.

According to Chinese medicine, exercise has two main health-promoting functions: First, it frees the flow of the qi, thus resolving liver depression. It the qi moves, then the blood and body fluids move. Therefore, exercise indirectly helps prevent and remedy blood stasis, damp accumulation, and phlegm nodulation. Secondly, exercise fortifies or strengthens the spleen and boosts the stomach. The spleen then produces more qi and blood on the one hand, while it promotes the excretion of waste products, including toxins, on the other.

One of my (Honora Lee Wolfe) clients recently reported that her chronic premenstrual breast distention is greatly reduced since she began regular aerobic exercise. Her report is not surprising. While exercise may not eradicate the root cause of breast diseases—stress and emotional imbalance—when combined with daily relaxation, it is very effective at coping with stress and relieving pent-up, stagnant qi. It is, therefore, an important part of preventive self-care and should not be overlooked.

Good Dietary Habits

In Chinese medicine, the function of the spleen and stomach are likened to a pot on a stove or still. The stomach receives the foods and liquids which then "rotten and ripen" like a mash in a fermentation vat. The spleen then cooks this mash and drives off (*i.e.,* transforms and upbears) the pure part. This pure part collects in the lungs to become the qi and in the heart to become the blood. In addition, Chinese medicine characterizes this transformation as a process of yang qi transforming yin substance. All the principles of Chinese dietary therapy, including what women with breast disease should and should not eat, are derived from these basic "facts."

We have seen that a healthy spleen is vitally important for keeping the liver in check and the qi freely flowing. In fact, nourishing or supplementing the spleen is a classically accepted method of treatment for liver disorders even when using herbal or acupuncture therapy.[28] We have also seen that the spleen is the root of qi and blood transformation and engenderment. Therefore, it is vitally important for women with breast disease to avoid foods which damage the spleen and to eat foods which promote a healthy spleen and qi and blood production.

Foods which damage the spleen

In terms of foods which damage the spleen, Chinese medicine begins with uncooked, chilled foods. If the process of digestion is likened to cooking, then cooking is nothing other than predigestion outside of the body. In Chinese medicine, it is a given that the overwhelming majority of all food should be cooked, *i.e.,* predigested. Although cooking may destroy some vital nutrients (in Chinese, qi), cooking does render the remaining nutrients much more easily assimilable. Therefore, even though some

---

[28] Lee, Miriam, *Insights of a Senior Acupuncturist: One Combination of Points Can Treat Many Diseases*, Blue Poppy Press, Boulder, CO, 1992, p. 17

nutrients have been lost, the net absorption of nutrients is greater with cooked foods than raw. Further, eating raw foods makes the spleen work harder and thus wears the spleen out more quickly. If one's spleen is very robust, eating uncooked, raw foods may not be so damaging, but we have already seen that many women's spleens are already weak because of their monthly menses overtaxing the spleen *vis à vis* blood production.

More importantly, chilled foods directly damage the spleen. Chilled, frozen foods and drinks neutralize the spleen's yang qi. The process of digestion is the process of warming all foods and drinks to 100° Fahrenheit within the stomach so that it may undergo transformation. If the spleen expends too much yang qi just warming the food up, then it will become damaged and weak. Therefore, all foods and liquids should be eaten and drunk at room temperature at the least and better at body temperature. The more signs and symptoms of spleen vacuity a woman presents, such as fatigue, chronically loose stools, undigested food in the stools, cold hands and feet, dizziness on standing up, and aversion to cold, the more closely she should avoid uncooked, chilled foods and drinks.

In addition, sugars and sweets directly damage the spleen. This is because sweet is the flavor which inherently "enters" the spleen. It is also an inherently dampening flavor according to Chinese medicine. This means that the body engenders or secretes fluids which gather and collect, transforming into dampness, in response to foods with an excessively sweet flavor. In Chinese medicine, it is said that the spleen is averse to dampness. Dampness is yin and controls or checks yang qi. The spleen's function is based on the transformative and transporting functions of yang qi. Therefore, anything which is excessively dampening can damage the spleen. The sweeter a food is, the more dampening and, therefore, more damaging it is to the spleen.

It is said in the *Nei Jing (The Inner Classic)* that the sweet flavor relaxes the liver. That is why people who are under stress typically crave sugars and sweets. Such sweets do *temporarily* relieve the feeling of being stressed, *i.e.*, the feeling of liver depression qi stagnation. However, since excessive sweets damage the spleen, indulging this craving typically results in most people's condition becoming even worse. Therefore, attention to avoiding sweets requires a great deal of care and self-discipline. For people under stress, sweets are as seductive and almost as addictive as alcohol to an alcoholic

Another group of foods which are dampening and, therefore, damaging to the spleen is what Chinese doctors call "sodden wheat foods." This means flour products such as bread and noodles. Wheat (as opposed to rice) is damp by nature. When wheat is steamed, yeasted, and/or refined, it becomes even more dampening. In addition, all oils and fats are damp by nature and, hence, may damage the spleen. The more oily or greasy a food is, the worse it is for the spleen.

Because milk contains a lot of fat, dairy products are another spleen-damaging, dampness-engendering food. This includes especially milk, butter, and cheese.[29]

If we put this all together, then ice cream is just about the worst thing a woman with a weak, damp spleen could eat. Ice cream is chilled, it is intensely sweet, and it is filled with fat. Therefore, it is a triple whamy when it comes to damaging the spleen. Likewise, pasta smothered in tomato sauce and cheese is a recipe for disaster. Pasta made from wheat flour is dampening, tomatoes are dampening, and cheese is dampening. In addition, what

---

[29] Some dairy products available in the West come from animals that have been injected with rBGH (recombinant bovine growth hormone). People who consume milk or other dairy products from cows injected with rBGH are at higher risk for breast and colon cancer due to its stimulation of insulin growth factor, a human growth hormone linked to higher rates of these two types of cancer. Reported in, "In The News", *Delicious Magazine*, June, 1996, p. 16, quoted from Epstein, Samuel, M.D., *International Journal of Health Services*, 1996, vol. 26

many women don't know is that a glass of fruit juice contains as much sugar as a candy bar, and, therefore, is also very damaging to the spleen and damp-engendering.

Below is a list of specific Western foods which are either un-cooked, chilled, too sweet, or too dampening and thus damaging to the spleen. Women with PMS should minimize or avoid these proportional to how weak and damp their spleen is.

Ice cream
Sugar
Candy, especially chocolate
Milk
Butter
Cheese
Margarine
Yogurt
Raw salads
Fruit juices

Juicy, sweet fruits, such as oranges, peaches, strawber-ries, and tomatoes
Fatty meats
Fried foods
Refined flour products
Yeasted bread
Nuts
Alcohol (which is essentially sugar)

If the spleen is weak and wet, one should also not eat too much at any one time. A weak spleen can be overwhelmed by a large meal, especially if any of the food is hard-to-digest. This then results in food stagnation which only impedes the free flow of qi all the more and further damages the spleen.

A clear, bland diet

In Chinese medicine, the best diet for the spleen and, therefore, by extension for most humans, is what is called a "clear, bland diet." This is a diet high in complex carbohydrates such as unrefined grains, especially rice, and beans. It is a diet which is high in *lightly cooked* vegetables. It is a diet which is low in fatty meats, oily, greasy, fried foods, and very sweet foods. However, it is not a completely vegetarian diet. Most women, in my experience do better eating one to two ounces of various types of meat two to four times per week. This animal flesh may be the highly popular but over-touted chicken and fish, but should also include some lean beef, pork, and lamb. Some fresh or cooked fruits may be eaten, but fruit juices should be avoided.

An added benefit of a diet high in grains, fruits, and vegetables is that these food have significant amounts of fiber in them. Studies suggest that women whose diets are high in fiber may have a reduced risk of breast cancer.[30]

In addition, women should make an effort to include tofu and tempeh, two soy foods now commonly available in North American grocery food stores, in their diet. Dr. Stephen Barnes, a professor of pharmacology and toxicology at the University of Alabama at Birmingham, has found that soy contains genistein, a plant compound that seems to block the cancer-stimulating process in the body.[31] Since we know that Asian women, who commonly eat soy foods as a regular part of their diet, have lower rates of breast cancer than women in other parts of the world, it seems to make sense to eat these foods regularly.

Warming spices such as nutmeg, cardamom, cinnamon, ginger, etc., may be eaten to good advantage in small amounts as long as there are no signs of stomach heat (see the patterns of disharmony listed above for these symptoms). They will tend to give a mild boost to qi movement, without the damaging and imbalancing effects of caffeine or heavy spicy foods. They can be included in the diet in judicious amounts.

Pearled barley and especially Chinese barley (Semen Coicis Lachryma Jobi or *Yi Yi Ren*) is also thought to protect the body from tumors.[32] It can be eaten cooked with other grains, made

---

[30] Castleman, Michael, "News About Breast Cancer That Could Save Your Life," *Family Circle*, May 13, 1997, p. 66.

[31] *Ibid.*, p. 66

[32] Mao-shing Ni, Ph.D., *The Tao of Nutrition*, Seven Star Communications, Santa Monica, CA, 1987, p. 79

into a soft-cooked porridge, or added to soups.

If you know of suspect that your spleen is weak, then you should eat several smaller meals rather than one or two large meals. In addition, because rice is 1) neutral in temperature, 2) it fortifies the spleen and supplements the qi, and 3) it eliminates dampness, rice should be the main or staple grain in the diet.

A few problem foods

There are a few "problem" foods which deserve special mention. The first of these is coffee. Most women with breast lumps or pain are aware of the connection between foods which contain xanthines (coffee, black teas, colas, chocolate) and the exacerbation of their symptoms.

Many women crave coffee for two reasons. First, coffee moves stuck qi. Therefore, if a woman suffers from liver depression qi stagnation, temporarily coffee will make her feel like her qi is flowing. Secondly, coffee transforms essence into qi and makes that qi temporarily available to the body. Therefore, women who suffer from spleen and/or kidney vacuity fatigue will get a temporary lift from coffee. They will feel like they have energy. However, once this energy is used up, they are left with a negative deficit. The coffee has transformed some of the essence stored in the kidneys into qi. This qi has been used, and now there is less stored essence. Since the blood and essence share a common source, coffee drinking may ultimately worsen any disease associated with blood or kidney vacuities. Since the kidneys are linked with the *chong* vessel and chronic breast diseases are associated with disharmonies of this vessel, coffee drinking can cause or aggravate breast diseases associated with the *chong* vessel.

A related problem food is chocolate. Chocolate is a combination of oil, sugar, and cocoa. We have seen that both oil and sugar are dampening and damaging to the spleen. Temporarily, the sugar will boost the spleen qi, but ultimately it will result in "sugar blues" or a hypoglycemic let-down. Cocoa stirs the life gate fire. The life gate fire is another name for kidney yang or kidney fire, and kidney fire is the source of sexual energy and desire. It is said that chocolate is the food of love, and from the Chinese medical point of view, that is true. Since chocolate stimulates kidney fire at the same time as it temporarily boosts the spleen, it does give one rush of yang qi. In addition, this rush of yang qi does move depression and stagnation, at least short-term. So it makes sense that some women with liver depression, spleen vacuity, and kidney yang debility might crave chocolate premenstrually. Despite the understandable cravings, quitting coffee, chocolate, and other caffeine substances altogether is probably the single most important dietary change a woman can make for herself.

Alcohol, when used occasionally and in small amounts, has the ability to relax the whole body and may relieve stress. However, alcohol is both damp and hot according to Chinese medical theory. It strongly moves the qi and blood. Therefore, persons with liver depression qi stagnation will feel temporarily better from drinking alcohol. However, the sugar in alcohol damages the spleen and engenders dampness which "gum up the works," while the heat (yang) in alcohol can waste the blood (yin) and aggravate or inflame depressive liver heat. Jin Zi-jiu, a famous 19th century physician, in the *Jin Zi-jiu Zhuan Ji (Jin Zi-jiu's Medical Contemplations)* states,

> Alcohol has a volatile nature which damages the Spirit and injures the blood. Its energy is hot and it leads to waste and decline. Alcohol first enters the gallbladder-liver where gallbladder fire first explodes. The *qi* loses its restraint and descension....The blood becomes unsettled and as a result, rebellious ascension with vomiting of blood can occur. Moreover, alcohol is damp as well as hot. dampness injures the spleen. This creates stagnant food and phlegm which easily overstuffs the *qi* mecha-

84

nism. In short... drinking injures the blood.[33]

Furthermore, several Western research studies have shown that as little as one drink a day may increase a woman's risk of breast cancer.[34] (A drink is defined as 12 ounces of beer, a cocktail with one shot of 80 proof liquor, or 4 ounces of wine.) On the other hand, other studies indicate that small amounts of alcohol may reduce the risk of heart disease, which kills far more women than breast cancer. However, in relationship to breast disease, it is the liver *qi* which is excessive and not free flowing. It is the liver *blood* which keeps liver *qi* relaxed, smooth, and free flowing. Therefore, similarly to caffeine, it is important to limit or curtail alcohol consumption in order not to waste or injure the blood.

Spicy, peppery, "hot" foods also move the qi, thereby giving some temporary relief to liver depression qi stagnation. However, like alcohol, the heat in spicy hot foods wastes the blood and can inflame yang.

In Chinese medicine, the sour flavor is inherently astringing and constricting. Sour flavored foods will only aggravate qi stagnation by astringing and restricting the qi and blood all the more. This is also why sweet and sour foods, such as orange juice and tomatoes are particularly bad for women with liver depression/spleen vacuity. The sour flavor astringes and constricts the qi, while the sweet flavor damages the spleen and engenders dampness.

In my (Bob Flaws) experience, diet sodas seem to contain something that damages the Chinese idea of the kidneys. They may not damage the spleen the same way that sugared sodas do, but that does not mean they are healthy and safe. I say that diet

---

[33] Jin Zi-jiu, *Jin Zi-jiu Zhang Ji (Jin Zi-jiu's Medical Contemplations)*, trans. by Michael Helme, *Timing and The Times*, Flaws, B., Chace, C., & Helme, M., Blue Poppy Press, Boulder, CO, 1986, p. 128

[34] *Op.cit*, Castleman, p. 66

sodas damage the kidneys since a number of my patients over the years have reported that, when they drink numerous diet sodas, they experience terminal dribbling, urinary incontinence, and low back and knee soreness and weakness. When they stop drinking diet sodas, these symptoms disappear. Taken as a group, in Chinese medicine, these are kidney vacuity symptoms. Since women with breast disease in their late 30s and throughout their 40s may suffer from concomitant kidney vacuity (along with liver depression and spleen vacuity), I typically recommend such women to steer clear of diet sodas so as not to weaken their kidneys any further or faster.

Green tea

Finally, there has been a great deal of research in recent years about the anti-carcinogenic qualities of green tea. Studies of people in Asia who drink regular and large quantities of green tea are known to have lower rates of many cancers.[35] This type of tea can be purchased in any health food store and even in many regular grocery stores. An organic version is even available. The tea is refreshing and has far less caffeine than black teas.

Drinking green tea can also be very helpful as a way to quit drinking coffee or colas without totally denying yourself any caffeine drinks at all. I will discuss the use of green tea again in the section medicinal teas under other self-help techniques.

Final words on diet

Eating is something everyone does every day. We have a great deal of choice in this area of our lives, and we can choose to use

---

[35] Jiang Qing-yun, *Shi Zhi Ben Cao (Food Treatment Materia Medica)*, Beijing Press, 1990, p. 175, and Zhang En-qin, editor-in-chief, *Health Preservation and Rehabilitation* from the Practical English-Chinese Library of Traditional Chinese Medicine, Publishing House of Shanghai College of Traditional Chinese Medicine, 1990, p. 286

food as a preventive tool to increase and improve or our health. Chinese medical wisdom offers us a way to make eating a strong preventive factor against cancer or any other type of disease for that matter. For further information on Chinese dietary therapy, we recommend *The Tao of Healthy Eating According to Chinese Medicine* by Bob Flaws, Blue Poppy Press, 1997, and *Prince Wen Hui's Cook: Chinese Dietary Therapy* by Bob Flaws and Honora Lee Wolfe, Paradigm Press, 1983. Other books on Chinese dietary therapy are included in the section called Learning More About Chinese Medicine in the back of this book.

Tobacco

Tobacco is not really a food, but it makes some sense to discuss tobacco smoking along with good diet. According to Chinese medicine, tobacco has a dry, bitter energy which damages the qi and attacks the lungs. The lungs, according to Chinese physiology, help keep the liver under control. If the lungs become vacuous and weak, the liver can easily become too strong. The lungs are also the mother of the kidneys, and it is the kidney water which keeps the liver nourished and moist, free from pathogenic heat.

Therefore, it is easy to see by the logic of Chinese medicine that smoking tobacco is not good for women with breast disease. However, the Chinese medicinal effects of tobacco are more complex than the above description might at first imply. When it says that tobacco damages the qi and attacks the lungs, this means that tobacco is extremely powerful at dispersing the qi. The lungs work in tandem with the liver in keeping the qi moving throughout the body. The lungs empower the pushing of the qi just as the heart empowers the pushing of the blood. The liver then permits the qi to move through the channels and vessels. Because of this close relationship, one way of relieving pent-up stagnant qi in the liver is to disperse the lung qi, and smoking tobacco does just that.

This means that smoking tobacco does give symptomatic relief from the feelings of liver depression qi stagnation. Temporarily, one feels more relaxed and more energized because of the free flow of qi. Unfortunately, this is only a quick fix, like eating sugar or drinking coffee or alcohol, and the long-term effects are absolutely the opposite. Hence one must keep smoking in order to maintain the same sense of qi flow and energy.

The good news is that ear acupuncture is extremely effective for helping to overcome and addiction to smoking. It can relieve the pent-up qi and stagnation in a healthy way, thus relieving the jitters and cravings associated with nicotine withdrawal.

Home Remedies for Breast Disease

In this chapter you will find a number of other home remedies and self-care techniques for both treating and preventing breast disease. Each of these suggested therapies is based on the logic of Chinese medicine in terms of the above-discussed disease mechanisms of both benign and malignant breast disease. Our suggestion is that you choose a couple of these to add to your self-care regime. The more serious or disturbing your breast disease, the more of these regimes you might want to do. In addition, you choice will also be affected by local availability of some of the ingredients.

Abdominal massage

Self-massage may sound strange to some women, but its efficacy for improving health has been known in Asia, and especially in Japan for centuries. Although there are self-massage regimes for the entire body, the abdomen is considered especially important. In Japanese massage, the abdomen, also sometimes called the *hara,* is the entire soft portion of the belly. It stretches from just below the diaphragm to the top of the pubic bone. In Asia this area is considered a person's vital center. Anatomically, it contains all the vital viscera and bowels of Oriental medicine except the heart and lungs. In traditional Japanese medicine, it is believed that a healthy abdomen is the sign of and key to health in general.

Traditionally, abdominal health is ascertained through palpation (touch). Pain, lumps and bumps, abnormal muscular tension, abnormal pulsation, and hyper- or hypotonicity may all be signs that the internal organs or tissues are imbalanced or diseased. A corollary of this is that, if pain or other abnormal findings in the abdomen are relieved, imbalance or disease of the viscera and bowels these reflect will simultaneously be relieved.

Happily, one can not only diagnose the balance and imbalance of the organs by palpating the abdomen but one can directly treat these with nothing more than pressure applied with one's own hands. Many famous Japanese therapists, such as Kiyoshi Kato and Naoichi Kuzome, treat the full range of human disease primarily through abdominal massage.

The liver, spleen, stomach, and intestines are of primary importance to health according to traditional Chinese medicine and all may be affected in a healthy way through abdominal self-massage. If the liver, spleen, stomach, and intestines function normally, abundant qi and blood will be produced. Likewise, the clear yang (the healthy qi of the body) will arise and the turbid yin (waste products) will descend for excretion and evacuation. This rise and descent is called the qi mechanism. A healthy qi mechanism insures that the qi and blood will travel unobstructedly in their proper directions and to their proper destinations, thus nourishing and empowering all the functions and tissues of the organism. When the qi mechanism and the stomach and intestines are functioning in a healthy way, neither qi, blood, dampness, phlegm, food, or fire will have an opportunity to become stagnant and thus give rise to disease.

Abdominal self-massage is one easy but nonetheless effective way to keep the qi and blood in the viscera flowing unobstructedly and the qi mechanism functioning normally. Although abdominal massage is often performed professionally in Japan by trained therapists, it is easy to do a simpler version oneself and is all the more effective when done on a daily basis.

Begin by lying on your back with your knees drawn up. If the feet are spread slightly apart, the knees can fall together in the center and hold themselves up without any further effort. Next, press with the flats of the fingers of both hands under the right ribs. Begin pressing as you exhale. Continue to press and exhale to a count of six. When inhaling, move the fingers down and over to the sides of the rib cage and exhale and press again. Do this three times until you wind up pressing under the floating ribs at your side. See the figure below for a visual image of this manuever.

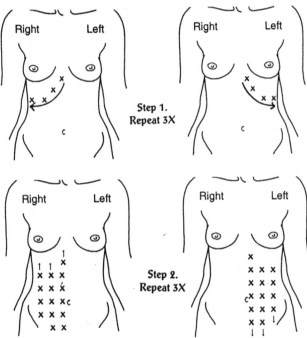

Next, go back to the midline beneath the ribs and repeat this sequence moving to the left in three exhalations. During this first pass over the hypochondrium, the pressure should not be too strong. Now repeat this entire sequence two more times, each time pressing a little harder.

At first, it is not uncommon to experience pain, resistance, or tension pressing on this area under the ribs, which is called the hypochondrium. This is a sign of congestion, mostly in the liver and gallbladder, which rule this area. As one continues over a period of weeks, this pain and tension will disappear and one's fingers will sink deeper under the ribs. This is quite important because it means that the liver's main function of governing the smooth dispersal of qi and blood is improving.

When the liver's smooth coursing and discharging function is healthy, peristalsis is normal and digestion is good. Also, one's mood will be even and light and one will have regular elimination and freedom from depression. Therefore, one can see that just this first movement promoting the free flow of the liver-gallbladder qi can have a deeply healing effect.

Next, position your hands on your lower right abdomen next to your pelvic bone. With each exhalation, press down for a count of six. As you inhale, move up the abdomen until finally your hands are beneath your ribs again. Make three passes up the abdomen on the right side. Anatomically, this follows the course of the ascending colon.

Then, beginning at the solar plexus, press down the midline to just above the pubic bone. Likewise, make three other lines down the left abdomen moving from the center out to the sides. These passes down the left abdomen follow the course of the descending colon. Repeat this entire sequence up the right and down the left sides of the abdomen three times, each time exerting a little more pressure.

Next, go back to any places where you felt special pain or resistance. As you exhale, exert pressure on these spots to the limits of your tolerance but without torturing yourself. Often the same spots or areas will be sore day after day. However, as you do this abdominal self-massage day by day, these areas will tend to become less sore and sensitive. Typically, in a relatively healthy person, after from two to four weeks of doing this regime daily, one's abdomen will become free from any such specially reactive areas. This signals that stagnations within the viscera and bowels have been relieved even before they may have given rise to any other signs and symptoms.

According to some doctors, if you find an actual lump or mass in the abdomen, besides having this checked by a primary health care professional, you should not press directly on the center of such a lump. Rather, you should search for a sore or sensitive spot on the edge or periphery of the lump. It is here that pressure should be exerted.[36]

Finally, return to the right hypochondrium and again press once three times out to the right and then from the solar plexus once three times out to the left. This concludes one's daily session of abdominal self-massage.

As mentioned above, after from two to four weeks of daily practice, the average person will find their abdomen has become painless and supple. This should be accompanied by better bowel movements, better appetite, and therefore better, more abundant energy. This entire procedure takes approximately 15-20 minutes. It can be performed directly upon arising or just before bed. After the abdomen becomes pain free and normalized, one can do the massage every other or every few days. However, if one does not take care of oneself, after some time, the pain, lumps, and tension may return and these are signs that one's imbalance has also reestablished itself.

In traditional Japanese medicine, it is felt that sensitive spots, lumps, and tension in the abdomen are precursors to more serious disease. A person may otherwise be symptom free but to many Japanese physicians, if there is some abnormality in the belly as diagnosed by palpation, there is some incipient disease process taking shape. Therefore, if you eliminate these abnormalities, you can abort such disease processes even before other signs and symptoms arise.

---

[36] Matsumoto, Kiiko, and Birch, Stephen, *Hara Diagnosis: Reflections on the Sea*, Paradigm Publications, Brookline, MA, 1988, p. 277-278

93

One cannot easily massage their entire body, but one *can* easily massage their abdomen. Since the abdomen is the root of the entire body, massaging it massages the root of all the rest. If the roots of a plant are healthy, the leaves and branches will likewise tend to flourish. Although abdominal self-massage appears simple, it is based on voluminous and profound theory. For those interested in reading more about the abdomen and its importance in Oriental medicine and also more about this type of massage, the reader is referred to *Hara Diagnosis: Reflections on the Sea* by Matsumoto and Birch.

Breast self-massage

While I (Honora Lee Wolfe) have been unable to find any written research about long-term effects of breast self-massage, massage of any area of the body will help to course and discharge the qi and move the blood in the local surface tissues. Because of this, massage has great potential positive effects for promoting breast health. In addition, in order for a woman to do this or any self-massage, she must stop and relax and take time for herself. This alone time is good for anyone's health. I strongly recommend some type of regular self-massage for all my clients and suggest that readers of this book give it a try.

Breast self-massage protocol

Begin by gently massaging any lumps within the breasts for 10 minutes. Then press and knead the center of the breastbone between the nipples. This is acupuncture point *Shan Zhong* (Conception Vessel 17). It regulates all the qi in the body and especially chest and breast qi. It also calms the spirit. Do this 100-200 times.

Next, knead the underarms with the tips of the middle fingers, first one underarm and then the other. Do this 100 times on each side.

94

Then push the breasts with both palms simultaneously. Push lightly from every side of the breasts towards the nipples for three to five minutes.

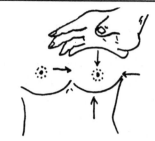

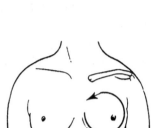

Fourth, rub the breasts lightly in circles. First rub the circles from the outside to the inside. Then reverse directions and rub from inside to outside. Do this until the breasts feel warm.

Fifth, rub the sides of the chest from the armpits downward to the center of the upper abdomen Do this until these areas feel warm.

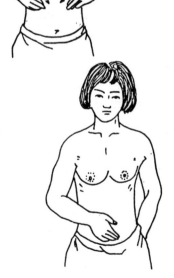

Finally, rub the abdomen in a circle in a clockwise direction around the navel for approximately five minutes.

The key to success with Chinese self-massage therapy is perseverance. Although a single massage may provide some symptomatic relief on that very day, it is repeated self-massage day after day which can make stable and lasting changes.

Magnet therapy

The Chinese have used magnet therapy since at least the Tang dynasty (618-907 CE). Placing magnets on the body is a safe and painless way of stimulating acupuncture points without inserting needles through the skin. Since magnets can be taped onto points and "worn" for days at a time, Chinese magnet therapy is able to provide easy, low cost, continuous treatment. Below are magnetic treatments for menstrual irregularities, including early, delayed, and erratic menstruation, excessive and scanty menstruation, lower abdominal pain occurring either before or at the onset of the period, and premenstrual breast distention and pain. Special adhesive magnets for stimulating acupuncture points, such as Accu-Band Magnets, Corimag, or Epaule Patch TDK Magnets, may be purchased from Oriental Medical Supply Co. located at 1950 Washington St., Braintree, MA 02184; Tel: (617) 331-3370 or 800-323-1839; Fax: (617) 335-5779. These range in strength from 400-9,000 gauss, the unit measuring magnetic strength. For the treatments below, one can try 400-800 gauss magnets.

Tape small body magnets over the following points with the south pole in contact with the skin if the condition is due to liver depression qi stagnation, depressive liver heat, or blood stasis. Place the north pole against the skin if the condition is due to spleen, liver, or kidney vacuities. Leave the magnets in place for three to five days at a time. Then remove for one day so that the body does not become habituated to this stimulation and reapply for another three to five days as needed.

Magnet therapy for premenstrual breast distention & pain and fibrocystic breasts

Tape small body magnets over the following points. Since most breast disease is at least locally a repletion or excess condition, tape the south sides in contact with the skin. Leave in place for three to five days. Then remove and take a rest for one day so as

96

to prevent the body from habituating to the stimulation. Then reapply as needed.

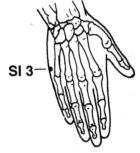

Hou Xi (Small Intestine 3): This point is located on the side of the hand below the little finger where the "heart line" meets the back of the hand. This point is known to have a very strong empirical effect on breast diseases due to counter-flowing qi in turn due to depression.

Ru Gen (Stomach 18): This point is located directly beneath the nipple in the fifth inter- costal space. It frees the flow of qi locally in the breasts and is used for a variety of breast diseases.

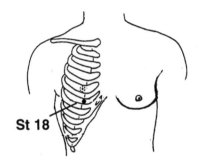

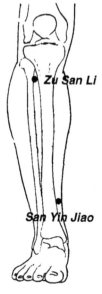

Zu San Li (Stomach 36): This point is located three inches below the lower, outside edge of the kneecap. It regulates the qi of the entire body and especially of the stomach channel which traverses the breasts. (See illustration on the next page.)

San Yin Jiao (Spleen 6): Point three inches above inner ankle bone shown at left.

If there are any cystic lumps, also tape a mag- net with the south side touching the skin directly over these.

Gan Shu (Bladder 18). This
point is located one and a
half inches lateral to the center
of the spine at the same level
as the lower edge of the ninth
thoracic vertebra. This point
connects directly with the liver
and is used to treat diseases due
to liver patterns of disharmony.

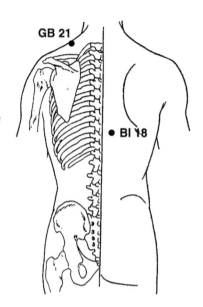

Jian Jing (Gallbladder 21):
This point is located at the
high point in the top center
of the trapezius or shoulder
muscle. It strongly downbears
upwardly counterflowing qi.

Chinese aromatherapy

In Chinese medicine, the qi is seen as a type of wind or vapor.
The Chinese character for qi shows wind blowing over a rice field.
In addition, smells are often referred to as a thing's qi. Therefore,
there is a close relationship between smells carried through the
air and the flow of qi in a person's body. Although aromatherapy
has not been a major part of professionally practiced Chinese
medicine for almost a thousand years, there is a simple
aromatherapy treatment which one can do at home which can
help alleviate premenstrual irritability, depression, nervousness,
anxiety, and insomnia due to liver depression qi stagnation. Since
most breast diseases are also, at least in part, due to liver
depression qi stagnation, aromatherapy can help the underlying
root mechanism if not immediately relieve the breast symptoms.
Since this is such an easy and enjoyable therapy to do, it can't
hurt.

In Chinese, *Chen Xiang* means "sinking fragrance." It is the name of Lignum Aquilariae Agallochae or Eaglewood. This is a frequent ingredient in Asian incense formulas. In Chinese medicine, Aquilaria is classified as a qi-rectifying medicinal. When used as a boiled decoction or "tea", Aquilaria moves the qi and stops pain, downbears upward counterflow and regulates the middle (*i.e.*, the spleen and stomach), and promotes the kidneys' grasping of the qi sent down by the lungs. I believe that the word sinking in this herb's name refers to this medicinal's down-bearing of upwardly counterflowing qi. Such upwardly counter-flowing eventually must accumulate in the heart, disturbing and causing restlessness of the heart spirit. When this medicinal wood is burnt and its smoke is inhaled as a medicinal incense, its downbearing and spirit-calming function is emphasized.

One can buy Aquilaria or *Chen Xiang* from Chinese herb stores in Chinatowns, Japantowns, or Koreatowns in major urban areas. One can also buy it from Chinese medical practitioners who have their own pharmacies. It is best to use the powdered variety. However, powder may be made by putting a small piece of this aromatic wood in a coffee grinder. It is also ok to use small bits of the wood if powder is not available. Next one needs to buy a roll of incense charcoals. Place one charcoal in non-flammable dish and light it with a match. Then sprinkle a few pinches of Aquilaria powder on the lit charcoal. As the smoke rises, breathe in deeply. This can be done on a regular basis one or more times per day during the premenstruum or on an as-needed basis by those suffering from restlessness, nervousness, anxiety, irritability, and depression. For those who experience premenstrual insomnia, one can do this "treatment" when lying in bed at night.

This Chinese aromatherapy with Lignum Aquilariae Agallochae is very cheap and effective. We know of no side effects or contra-indications.

Flower therapy

People have been bringing other people flowers for millennia to help them feel good. In Chinese medicine, there is actually a practice of flower therapy. Because the beauty of flowers bring most people joy and because joy is the antidote to the other four or seven negative emotions of Chinese medicine, flowers can help promote the free and easy flow of qi. It is said in Chinese medicine that, "Joy leads to relaxation (in the flow of qi)", and relaxation is exactly what the doctor ordered in cases of premenstrual liver depression qi stagnation. As Wu Shi-ji wrote in the Qing dynasty, "Enjoying flowers can divert a person from their boredom and alleviate suffering caused by the seven affects (or emotions)."

However, there is more to Chinese flower therapy than the beauty of flowers bringing joy. Flower therapy also includes aromatherapy. A number of Chinese medicinals come from plants which have flowers used in bouquets. For instance, Chrysanthemum flowers (*Ju Hua*, Flos Chrysanthemi Morifolii) are used to calm the liver and clear depressive heat rising to the upper body. The aroma of Chrysanthemum flowers thus also has a salutary, relaxing, and cooling effect on liver depression and depressive heat. Rose (*Mei Gui Hua,* Flos Rosae Rugosae) is used in Chinese medicine to move the qi and quicken the blood. Smelling the fragrance of Roses also does these same things. Other flowers used in Chinese medicine to calm the spirit and relieve stress and irritability are Lily, Narcissus, Lotus flowers, Orchids, and Jasmine. And further, taking a smell of a bouquet of flowers promotes deep breathing, and this, in turn, relieves pent up qi in the chest at the same time as it promotes the flow of qi downward via the lungs.

Thread moxibustion

Thread moxibustion refers to burning extremely tiny cones or "threads" of aged Oriental mugwort directly on top of certain acupuncture points. When done correctly, this is a very simple and effective way of adding yang qi to the body without causing a burn or scar.

To do thread moxa, one must first purchase the finest grade Japanese moxa wool. This is available from Oriental Medical Supplies mentioned above under magnet therapy. It is listed under the name Gold Direct Moxa. Pinch off a very small amount of this loose moxa wool and roll it lightly between the thumb and forefinger. What you want to wind up with is a very loose, very thin thread of moxa smaller than a grain of rice. It is important that this thread not be too large or too tightly wrapped.

Next, rub a very thin film of Tiger Balm or Temple of Heaven Balm on the point to be moxaed. These are camphored Chinese medical salves which are widely available in North American health food stores. Be sure to apply nothing more than the thinnest film of salve. If such a Chinese medicated salve is not available, then wipe the point with a tiny amount of vegetable oil. Stand the thread of moxa up perpendicularly directly over the point to be moxaed. The oil or balm should provide enough stickiness to make the thread stand on end. Light the thread with a burning incense stick. As the thread burns down towards the skin, you will feel more and more heat. Immediately remove the burning thread when you begin to feel the burning thread go from hot to too hot. *Do not burn yourself.* It is better to pull the thread off too soon than too late. In this case, more is not better than enough. (If you do burn yourself, apply some *Ching Wan Hong* ointment. This is a Chinese burn salve which is available at Chinese apothecaries and is truly wonderful for treating all sorts of burns. It should be in every home's medicine cabinet.)

Having removed the burning thread and extinguished it between your two fingers, repeat this process again. To make this process go faster and more efficiently, one can roll a number of threads before starting the treatment. Each time the thread burns down close to the skin, pinch it off the skin and extinguish it *before* it starts to burn you. If you do this correctly, your skin will get red and hot to the touch but you will not raise a blister. Because everyone's skin is different, the first time you do this, only start out with three or four threads. Each day, increase this number until you reach nine to twelve threads per treatment.

This treatment is especially effective for women in their late 30s and throughout their 40s whose spleen and kidney yang qi has already become weak and insufficient. Since this treatment actually adds yang qi to the body, this type of thread moxa fortifies the spleen and invigorates the kidneys, warming yang and boosting the qi. Because the stimuli is not that strong at any given treatment, it must be done every day for a number of days. For women who suffer from pronounced premenstrual fatigue, loose stools, cold hands and feet, low or no libido, and low back or knee pain accompanied by frequent nighttime urination along with premenstrual breast distention or fibrocystic breasts, I recommend beginning this moxibustion just before ovulation, around day 10 in the cycle. It should then be repeated every day up through day one of the period and then suspended. It can be done for several months in a row, but should not usually be done continuously throughout the year, day in and day out.

There is one main point which should be moxaed using this supplementing technique. It is:

Guan Yuan (Conception Vessel 4) I recommend visiting a local professional acupuncturist so that they can teach you how to do this technique safely and effectively and to show you how to locate this point accurately.

● Guan Yuan

In Chinese medicine, this technique is considered a longevity and health preservation technique. It is great for those people whose yang qi has already begun to decline due to the inevitable aging process. It should not be done by people with ascension of hyperactive liver yang, liver fire, or depressive liver heat. *If there is any doubt about whether this technique is appropriate for you, please see a professional practitioner for a diagnosis and individualized recommendation.*

Light therapy

Light therapy, more specifically sunbathing or heliotherapy, is one of Chinese medicine's health preservation and longevity practices. Sunlight is considered the most essential yang qi in nature. Li Shi-zhen, one of the most famous Chinese doctors of the late Ming dynasty (1368-1644 CE) wrote, "*Tai yang* (literally, supreme yang but a name for the sun) is true fire." As he pointed out, "Without fire, heaven is not able to engender things, and without fire, people are not able to live." Because the back of the human body is yang (as compared to the front which is more yin), exposing the back to sunlight is a good way of increasing one's yang qi.

As we have seen above, most women's yang qi begins to decline by around 35 years of age. In women over 35 years of age, most premenstrual fatigue, loose stools, lack of strength, poor memory, lack of concentration, poor coordination, decline in or lack of libido, low back and knee soreness and weakness, increased nighttime urination, and cold hands and feet are due to this decline first in the yang qi of the spleen and later in the yang qi of the spleen and kidneys. When many women say they are depressed, what they mean in Chinese medical terms is that they are extremely fatigued. In such cases, sunbathing can help supplement the yang qi of the body, thereby strengthening the spleen and/or kidneys.

103

However, because the yang qi is also the motivating force which pushes the qi, increasing yang qi can also help resolve depression and move stagnation. Cao Ting-dong, a famous doctor of the Qing dynasty (1644-1911 CE) wrote:

> Sitting with the back exposed directly to the sun, the back may get warmed. This able to make the entire body harmonious and smoothly flowing. The sun is the essence of *tai yang* and its light strengthens the yang qi of the human body.

In Chinese medicine, whenever the words harmonious and smoothly flowing are used together, they refer to the flow of qi and blood. Hence sun-bathing can help course the liver and rectify the qi as well as fortify the spleen and invigorate the kidneys.

It has been said that sunlight is good for every disease except skin cancer. In particular, vitamin D derived from sunbathing may help prevent both breast and colon cancer.[37] On the other hand, as we now know, overexposure to the sun can cause skin cancer due to sunlight damaging the cells of the skin. Therefore, one should be careful not to get too much sun and not to get burnt. In Chinese medicine, sun-bathing should be done between the hours of 8-10 AM. One should only sun-bathe between 11 AM-1 PM in winter in temperate, not tropical, latitudes.

It is interesting to note that some Western researchers are coming to understand that exposure to light also plays a role in many women's PMS.

Dandelion

Dandelion has long been known in China as an effective medicinal for treating breast diseases. Dandelion, Herba Taraxaci Mongolici Cum Radice (*Pu Gong Ying*), clears heat, nourishes yin,

---

[37] "Can Sunshine Save Your Life?", *Newsweek*, Dec. 30,1991, p. 56

and resolves fire toxins. It rectifies the qi, disperses swelling, and scatters nodulation. It is thought to have a special tropism for the chest and breast area and is often used to relieve the pain and swelling of mastitis and to promote lactation. It is also considered one of the special anti-cancer Chinese medicinals. Dandelion is also a common Western herb and can usually be purchased in bulk in health food stores. There are several ways in which this medicinal can be used as a home remedy.

Dandelion Wine

Herbal wines and liqueurs are an ancient, commonly used method of administering medicine. Alcohol, in small amounts, can scatter cold, supplement and move the qi and blood, revitalizes the spirit, and is also an effective medium for getting medicine into the blood quickly. However, if alcohol consumption typically aggravates a woman's breast condition, then drinking dandelion wine is probably not a good idea.

Dandelion wine resolves toxins, disperses swelling, scatters nodulation, and stops pain. It is prescribed for the treatment of breast swelling and pain and breast abscesses. Breast abscesses or mastitis are usually a hot condition, and alcohol's nature is hot. In Chinese medicine, we usually treat hot conditions with cold medicinals. So using a wine or alcohol-based medicine looks at first contradictory. However, dandelion's nature is cold. In this case, dandelion's cold nature overrides the heat of alcohol to clear heat and resolve toxins.

To make this "wine", take a large handful of dandelion and crush it in a mortar. Stir the resulting mash into a cupful of brandy, dry sherry, sake, or vodka and let stand for at least a few hours or up to several days, covered so that the alcohol does not evaporate. Strain out the dregs and drink a small teacupful each day. This can actually be made fresh each day, since it does not require long time to tincture.

105

This wine or tincture can also be massaged into the breasts or used as a compress over inflamed lumps. In that case, add a few pinches of myrrh (Resina Myrrhae, *Mo Yao*) and warm the wine before use. For more information on making and using Chinese medicinal wines, see *Chinese Medicinal Wines and Elixirs* by Bob Flaws also available from Blue Poppy Press.

Dandelion tea

Simple medicinal teas that are made fresh are a very convenient way to take herbal medicinals at home. Unlike Chinese medicinal decoctions having eight to 20 ingredients and a notoriously foul taste, these teas can be made fresh in just a few minutes and drunk as a daily beverage. They can even be mixed with black or green teas and a very little white or brown sugar.

Dandelion tea can be made simply by pouring boiling water over a small handful of dandelion. For a slightly more complex beverage, one could mix the dandelion with a small amount of green tea, and/or a small amount of green orange peel (Pericarpium Citri Reticulatae Viride, *Qing Pi*). The green tea will add to the heat-clearing effect of the beverage. The green orange peel will add to its qi-moving and rectifying effect.

For more information on simple Chinese medicinal tea formulas, see *Chinese Medicine Teas: Simple Proven Folk Formulas for Common Diseases and Promoting Health* by Zong Xiao-fan and Gary Liscum from Blue Poppy Press.

Dandelion porridge or congee

In many parts of China, medicinal herbs are mixed with stews and porridges to make herbal food dishes. Usually eaten for breakfast, medicinal porridges combine specific grains, vegetables, meats, eggs, and Chinese herbs. Like medicinal teas and wines, porridges can be used either remedially or preventively and are an easy way to ingest one's "medicine".

106

When making a porridge with dandelion, rice is the most commonly used grain. Take one cup rice, 6 cups water, and 30 grams (about 2 ounces) of dandelion. Put in a crock pot and set on low heat. Cook for 6-8 hours. This will make a medium thick porridge and can be made thinker or thinner depending upon the water to rice ratio. Eat with a very small amount of sugar or salt. This porridge clears heat and resolves toxins, disperses swelling and scatters nodulation and is often used for nursing mothers to treat or prevent mastitis. Just like in the dandelion tea, it is possible to add Chinese green orange peel. This second herb will help to course the liver, rectify the qi, and disperse swelling.

If you are unable to find dandelion or orange peel at a local health food store, you can get these herbs and the others discussed below directly from:

China Herb Co.
165 W. Queen Lane
Philadelphia, PA 19144
Tel: 215-843-5864 Fax: 215-849-3338 Orders: 800-221-4372

...ese Herbal Congees & Teas

other simple Chinese herbal congees and teas.
the spleen and eliminate dampness or they
d rectify the qi. In some cases, they do both
ngs.

...ruation-regulating Tea

regulate menstruation by coursing the liver
qi, quickening the blood and transforming
is also good for promoting the health of the
nnection between the liver and the breasts
he breasts. It is made by taking 9 grams of
ae Rugosae, *Mei Gui Hua*), 9 grams of rose

107

hips (Fructus Rosae Chinensis, *Yue Ji Hua*), and 3 grams of green tea. Grind these three ingredients into coarse powder and steep in boiling water for 10 minutes. Drink the resulting tea warm throughout the day from ovulation through menstruation if you have a tendency to painful menstruation accompanied by premenstrual breast distention and pain. You can also make this tea without the rose hips.

Rose & Buddha's Hand Tea

This tea also uses rose flowers. Take 6 grams of Flos Rosae Rugosae (*Mei Gui Hua*) and 10 grams of finger citron (Fructus Citri Sacrodactylis, *Fo Shou* or Buddha's Hand fruit) and steep in boiling water for 5-10 minutes. Drink warm at any time of the day. This tea courses the liver and rectifies the qi as well as quickens the blood and transforms stasis.

Motherwort Tea

This tea is also good if a woman has a tendency for blood stasis with painful menstruation. It is made by steeping 20 grams of motherwort (Herba Leonuri Heterophylli, *Yi Mu Cao*) with one gram of green tea in boiling water for 10 minutes. It also should be drunk from ovulation through the menstrual period.

Malted Barley & Hawthorne Fruit Tea

This tea is made from 10 grams of malted barley (Fructus Germinatus Hordei Vulgaris, *Mai Ya*), 3 grams of hawthorne berries (Fructus Crataegi, *Shan Zha*), and a little brown sugar to taste. Add these three ingredients to water and boil for a short time. Discard the dregs and drink the resulting liquid freely throughout the day. This tea courses the liver and rectifies the qi especially in the breasts. It also helps quicken the blood and disperse nodulations. However, it should not be drunk by lactating mothers, since malted barley is the main Chinese medicinal for stopping lactation. It stops lactation because it so strongly disperses the qi and, therefore, blood and body fluids in the breasts.

Licorice & Orange Peel Tea

If spleen vacuity is more of an issue than liver depression qi stagnation or blood stasis, than the following two herb tea may be just right for you. Take 10 grams of dried orange peel (Pericarpium Citri Reticulatae, *Chen Pi*) and 5 grams of licorice root (Radix Glycyrrhizae Uralensis, *Gan Cao*). Steep these in boiling water for 5-10 minutes and drink warm after meals, three times each day. Do not use this tea if your blood pressure is high, since licorice can raise blood pressure. In actual fact, most women with spleen vacuity weakness have low blood pressure.

Orange Peel Tea

If you have large or small, well-defined, hard, rubbery nodulations in your breasts, Chinese doctors would probably say you have phlegm nodulation as at least part of your TCM pattern. If you tend to have lots of lung or nasal mucus or even excessive white vaginal discharge, this confirms that phlegm is part of your pattern even more. In that case, the following tea may help eliminate phlegm dampness. Take 2 grams of dried orange peel (Pericarpium Citri Reticulatae, *Chen Pi*) and 2 grams of green tea. Steep in boiling water for 5-10 minutes and drink especially after meals.

Another version of this tea is to use orange peel and three Chinese red jujube fruits (Fructus Zizyphi Jujubae, *Da Zao*). Steep these in boiling water and drink often throughout the day.

Dry Ginger Congee

This Chinese medicinal porridge is good if your spleen has become weak accompanied by cold hands and feet, a cold nose, and a tendency to loose stools. Cook 5 grams of dry ginger (dry

Rhizoma Zingiberis, *Gan Jiang*) in 100 grams of white rice and three times more water than if you were cooking rice to eat ordinarily. Eat this every morning on an empty stomach.

Fennel Congee

This congee can be good if you have liver depression and a cold, weak spleen. In that case, you probably have premenstrual breast distention, painful periods, and a lot of bloating and gas after meals. Take 5 grams of fennel seed (Fructus Foeniculi Vulgaris, *Xiao Hui Xiang*), 50 grams of white rice, and just a tiny little bit of brown sugar. Stir-fry the fennel until it turns yellow before cooking it with the rice in three times more water than usual. Eat warm one time per day in the evening before going to bed.

Rice & Coix Congee

This congee supplements the spleen and eliminates dampness. In addition, coix or Job's tears barley is believed to have specific cancer-preventing properties. Take 100 grams of white rice, 50 grams of coix (Semen Coicis Lachryma-jobi, *Yi Yi Ren*), and 10 Chinese red jujubes (Fructus Zizyphi Jujubae, *Da Zao*) and make into porridge with a suitable amount of water. Eat this one time each day for a long time.

Poria Congee

Poria is another spleen-supplementing, dampness-eliminating Chinese medicinal which is also believed to be a specific cancer-preventing herb or food. Take 50 grams of powdered poria (Sclerotium Poriae Cocos, *Fu Ling*) and 100 grams of white rice. Cook the rice in water into porridge. Towards the end, stir in the poria powder and cook a while longer. Then eat regularly.

Dioscorea Congee

Chinese wild yam is believed to supplement both the spleen and kidneys at the same time without aggravating any evil heat in the body. Since many women develop spleen-kidney vacuity as they age, this congee is not a bad one to eat on a regular basis. To make it, take 50grams of powdered Chinese wild yam root (Radix Dioscoreae Oppositae, *Shan Yao*) and cook with 100g of white rice the same as in the preceding congee. Eat this regularly.

As we mentioned above, many Western researchers believe that a number of breast problems are due to an imbalance in estrogen-progesterone production which often crops up as the ovaries age and cease to function optimally. In that case, during the second half of the menstrual cycle, from ovulation to the onset of menstruation, progesterone is too little and, therefore, estrogen appears to be too much. Recently, a number of Western pharmaceutical companies have been selling extracts of wild yam as a treatment for progesterone deficiency. Chinese doctors have been prescribing this herb to perimenopausal women for 2,000 years.

Compresses

A compress is made by dipping a towel in a hot decoction or infusion of a medicinal tea. The towel is wrung out and placed over the area to be treated. Heat in general promotes the flow of qi and blood in any area it is applied to. If one adds some medicinals which also help move the qi and quicken the blood, this effect can be made even stronger. In Chinese medicine, there are numerous compress recipes for helping disperse swelling and heat from the breasts and to improve the flow of qi and blood through the breasts. Above we saw how we could apply dandelion wine to the breasts as either a massage liniment or a compress. Below is another compress recipe specifically for the breasts.

Take Radix Trichosanthis Kirlowii (*Tian Hua Fen*), 15g, Bulbus Allii (*Xiong Bai*), 9g, and Resina Myrrhae (*Mo Yao*), 9g. Boil these three ingredients in half wine and half water for 30 minutes. Discard the dregs and use as a compress for sore, swollen breasts and a feeling of tightness and constriction in the chest premenstrually.

Obviously, you are not going to have time to do all of the above self-care treatments, nor do you need to. As mentioned above, simply chose the couple or several which suit your needs and time the best. If you experience *any* side or unwanted effects from any of these recommendations, stop immediately and seek advice from a qualified professional practitioner of Chinese medicine. Remember, the goal of Chinese medical treatment is healing without side effects. So please don't think that any side effects are acceptable. In addition, you local professional practitioner should be able to teach you even more self-care treatments and tips to help insure healthy breasts.

Professional Therapies

While all these self-care treatments are useful and will improve the situation of any woman experiencing breast pain, distention, or lumps, they may not be enough. If symptoms persist, or if lumps are already present, professionally administered therapies may be necessary for quicker and greater long-term remission of symptoms. Here let us say again that successful treatment can take place *at any point in this process*, no matter what the symptoms, if a woman has the motivation and will.

Professionally administered Chinese medicine is definitely effective in the treatment of the majority of breast diseases. Several recent studies available in acupuncture and Chinese medical journals show excellent results in the treatment of breast neoplasms with the use of acupuncture or Chinese herbal medicine. A study of 128 women with fibrocystic breast disease and benign breast lumps showed a 95.31% cure rate using herbal medicine.[38] In a study of 500 cases of hyperplasia (lumps) of the breast treated by acupuncture, there was a 95.71% effective rate with only one course of 10 treatments. These results were better than the control group which was treated with a combination of Chinese herbal medicine and Western drug therapy.[39] In another experimental study on mice with breast tumors, a combination of

---

[38] Mi Yang, MD, "The Treatment of Benign Breast Disease", *Hunan Journal of Traditional Chinese Medicine*, #1, 1993, p. 47

[39] Chang, Yung-hsien, Haw, Dou-mong, and Hung, Yu-tse, "Effect of Irradiation and Moxibustion on Mice Bearing Breast Tumor", *Fourth International Congress of Chinese Medicine,* University of San Francisco, CA, July 29-31, 1988.

radiation therapy and moxibustion was used.[40] The group of mice treated with this combination of therapies showed the longest survival rate of the four different groups tested.[41] Another study of treating benign breast lumps in 24 women reported a 91.7% cure and improvement rate.[42] Most American practitioners will want to administer a combination of both herbal and acupuncture therapy, although either may be effective depending upon the case. For readers interested in more information on Chinese breast disease research, see the next chapter which is composed abstracts of recent research on breast disease from Chinese medical journals.

Herbal medicine or acupuncture?

Acupuncture and Chinese herbal medicine are the two main modalities or treatments of professional Chinese medicine. Most Western practitioners are primarily licensed as acupuncturists and may or may not also practice Chinese herbal medicine. In general, the more there are pathological changes in the tissue itself, the more emphasis should be placed on Chinese herbal medicine as opposed to acupuncture. However, our 20 years of clinical experience and the Chinese literature suggests that, when it comes to breast diseases, acupuncture is an extremely part of an overall treatment plan. Chinese herbal medicine alone may or may not get completely satisfactory results, while acupuncture typically gets very startling and immediate results. As we will see below, acupuncture can be used to remedially treat

---

[40] Moxibustion is a treatment procedure in Chinese medicine whereby an herbal ingredient, *Artemesiae Vulgaris Sinensis*, is burned over, under, on, or around an acupuncture point. This therapy is usually used to warm and tonify the organ or channel being treated.

[41] Guo Chengjie, "Effects of Acupuncture in the Treatment of 500 Cases of Hyperplasia of Breast", *Chinese Acupuncture & Moxibustion*, Vol. 6, No.4, August, 1986, pp.2-4

[42] Hou Jian, MD, "Herbal Treatment of Breast Hyperplasia", *Shandong Journal of Traditional Chinese Medicine*, #5, 1993, p. 24-25.

already occurring breast diseases as well as provide preventive care.

If a woman has developed breast cancer, probably the best treatment is a combination of traditional Chinese and modern Western medicines. By the time an imbalance has degenerated to cancer, traditional Chinese medicine by itself is typically not fast enough. Western medicine, although heroic and quick, often also causes side-effects. Happily, these side-effects can usually be treated very well with Chinese medicine. These days, more and more patients and physicians alike are opting for lumpectomies whenever possible followed by radiation and/or chemotherapy. Chinese herbal medicine can be taken before surgery to minimize bleeding and promote quicker recuperation. Chinese herbal medicine can be used to minimize the negative effects of radiation. And Chinese herbal medicine can also be taken during and after chemotherapy to minimize and treat its side effects usually quite effectively, including nausea, fatigue, anemia, and even hair loss. *The Treatment of Cancer by Integrated Chinese-Western Medicine* by Zhang Dai-zhao presents a very clear, step by step methodology for combining Chinese and Western medicines in the treatment of breast cancer.[43]

Women who have already been treated by Western medicine alone for breast cancer should also consider that Western medicine rarely treats the underlying reasons for the development of cancer in the first place. These underlying disease mechanisms may persist after surgery, radiation, and/or chemotherapy and this explains why cancer often recurs. These heroic and swift therapies may give a woman a much needed respite, but she should not be fooled into thinking that they have aborted the energetic process at the root of her problem. Traditional Chinese medicine, on the other hand, typically can identify and

---

[43] Zhang Dai-zhao, *The Treatment of Cancer by Integrated Chinese-Western Medicine*, trans. by Zhang Ting-liang & Bob Flaws, Blue Poppy Press, Boulder, CO, 1988, currently out of print.

treat these root causes, especially if a woman is willing to be directly involved in her own self-care. Such treatment usually is a life-time process. As Dr. Zhang says,

> ...perseverance in prolonged and active integrated therapy is one important step to consolidate and enhance the therapeutic effect and prevent recurrence. Malignant tumors are characterized by their rapid growth and their tendency to reoccur and metastasize. Due to the fact that there is no satisfactory radical therapy for late stage cancers, it is more important that doctors assume a responsible attitude in order to maintain a long-term relationship and to offer (their) knowledge of preventing and treating cancerous conditions, thus encouraging patients to continue long-term treatment. It should never be assumed that when the symptoms are relieved after treatments such as surgery, radiation, chemotherapy, or the internal ingestion of herbal ingredients for a period of time that the cancerous condition has been (completely) corrected and that therapy should be suspended.[44]

What is acupuncture?

Acupuncture primarily means the insertion of extremely thin, sterilized, stainless steel needles into specific points on the body where Chinese doctors have known for centuries there are special concentrations of qi and blood. Therefore, these points are like switches or circuit breakers for regulating and balancing the flow of qi and blood over the channel and network system we described above. As we have seen, there really is no breast disease if there is not also liver depression, and liver depression means that the qi is stagnant. Because the qi is depressed and stagnant, it is not flowing when and where it should. Instead it counterflows or vents itself to areas of the body where it shouldn't be, attacking other organs and body tissues and making them dysfunctional.

---

[44] *Ibid.*, p. 135-136

Therefore, breast disease typically includes many signs and symptoms associated with lack of, errroneous, or counterflow qi. Since acupuncture's forte is the regulation and rectification of the flow of qi (and, thus secondarily, the blood), it can be an effective treatment mode for correcting less serious breast diseases. In that case, insertion of acupuncture needles at various points in the body moves stagnant qi in the liver and leads the qi to flow in its proper directions and amounts.

As a generic term, acupuncture also includes several other methods of stimulating acupuncture points, thus regulating the flow of qi in the body. The main other modality is called moxibustion. This means the warming of acupuncture points mainly by burning dried, aged Oriental mugwort on, near, or over acupuncture points. The purpose of this warming treatment are to 1) even more strongly stimulate the flow of qi and blood, 2) add warmth to areas of the body which are too cold, and 3) add yang qi to the body to supplement a yang qi deficiency. Other acupuncture modalities are to apply suction cups over points, to massage the points, to prick the points to allow a drop or two of blood to exit, to apply Chinese medicinals to the points, to apply magnets to the points, and to stimulate the points by either electricity or laser.

What is a typical acupuncture treatment for breast disease like?

In China, treatments for breast diseases which are cyclic with the menstruation are administered starting as soon as possible from the onset of any signs or symptoms each month. Once the symptoms appear, treatment is given every other day or as often as possible through the first day of menstruation or until the symptoms disappear. This regime is then repeated again the next month. However, if the treatment has been correct and if the woman has been following her practitioner's advice about diet, exercise, lifestyle, and relaxation, then her symptoms should lessen each month. This means that she should need less and less treatments each month.

When the woman comes for her appointment, the practitioner will ask her what her main symptoms are, will typically look at her tongue and its fur, and will feel the pulses at the radial arteries on both wrists. Then, they will ask the woman to lie down on a treatment table. Based on their Chinese pattern discrimination, the practitioner will select anywhere from one to eight or nine points to be needled.

The needles used today are ethylene oxide gas sterilized disposable needles. This means that they are used one time and then thrown away, just like a hypodermic syringe in a doctor's office. However, unlike relatively fat hypodermic needles, acupuncture needles are hardly thicker than a strand of hair. The skin over the point is disinfected with alcohol and the needle is quickly and deftly inserted somewhere typically between one quarter and a half inch. In some few cases, a needle may be inserted deeper than that, but most needles are only inserted relatively shallowly. Usually the needles are left in place from 10-20 minutes. After this, the needles are withdrawn and thrown away. *Thus there is absolutely no chance for infection from another patient.*

How are the points selected?

The points an acupuncturist chooses to needle each treatment are selected either on the basis of Chinese medical theory, by palpation of the local area and related channels, and the known clinical effects of certain points. Since there are different schools or styles of acupuncture, point selection tends to vary from practitioner to practitioner. However, let me present a fairly typical case from the point of view of the dominant style of acupuncture in the People's Republic of China.

Let's say the woman's main complaints are premenstrual breast distention and pain but no lumps or cystic tissue, irritability, fatigue, and loose stools. Her tongue is fat and pale with thin, slightly slimy, white fur, and her pulse is fine and bowstring. Her Chinese pattern discrimination is premenstrual breast distention and pain, easy anger, and fatigue due to liver depression and spleen vacuity. This is a very commonly encountered Chinese pattern of disharmony.

The treatment principles necessary for remedying this case are to course the liver and rectify the qi, fortify the spleen and supplement the qi. In addition, because breast distention and pain are major complaints, the practitioner will add the treatment principles of loosen the chest and free the flow in the breasts. In order to accomplish these aims, the practitioner might select the following points:

Tai Chong (Liver 3)
San Yin Jiao (Spleen 6)
Zu San Li (Stomach 36)
Ru Gen (Stomach 18)
Shan Zhong (Conception Vessel 17)
Pi Shu (Bladder 20)
Wei Shu (Bladder 21)
Ah shi or tender points as needed

In this case, *Tai Chong* courses the liver and resolves depression, moves and rectifies the qi. Since liver depression qi stagnation is the main disease mechanism causing this woman's PMS, this is the main or ruling point in this treatment. Since this woman's easy anger or irritability stems from liver depression, this point also eliminates the source of this woman's vexation.

San Yin Jiao is chosen to further course the liver at the same time as it fortifies the spleen. It does both these things because both the liver and spleen channels cross at this point. In addition, this point is known to be empirically effective for most genitourinary and reproductive diseases. In Chinese medicine, it is said to possess a menstruation-regulating effect.

Zu San Li is the most powerful point on the stomach channel. Because the stomach is yang and the spleen is yin and because the stomach and spleen share a mutually "exterior/interior" relationship, stimulating *Zu San Li* can bolster the spleen with yang qi from the stomach which usually has plenty. In addition, the stomach channel traverses the breasts and, therefore, needling this point can regulate or rectify the qi in the breasts.

Ru Gen is also a point on the stomach channel. However, it is located just under the breasts and is a main local point for freeing and regulating the flow of qi through the breasts. Likewise, *Shan Zhong*, which is located at the level of the nipples on the chest bone between the breasts, is also a local point for freeing the flow of qi in the chest and breasts. This point is a special point for regulating the flow of qi in the entire body, but especially in the chest. It also helps calm the spirit and provide emotional relief.

Pi Shu and *Wei Shu* are both points on the back associated with the spleen and stomach respectively. They directly connect with this viscus and bowel and can supplement weakness and deficiencies in these two organs. In particular, this woman's fatigue and loose stools both stem from spleen vacuity, and these two points are known to empirically address both of these complaints.

Ah shi points are acupuncture points that are located by the acupuncturist palpating the channels and local areas which are affected by a person's disorder. Any locations or areas which are tender to pressure, raised or hard, sunken, or with a variation in the normal temperature or texture of the skin, may be chosen for treatment either with needles or other techniques such as moxibustion. In order to normalize the flow of qi in a specific area of the body, *ah shi* points can be very important in the efficacy of treatment, especially where pain and distention are among the person's symptoms.

Thus this combination of points addresses this woman's Chinese pattern discrimination and her major complaints of breast distention and soreness, irritability, and fatigue and loose stools. It remedies both the underlying disease mechanism and addresses certain key symptoms in a very direct and immediate way. Hence it provides symptomatic relief *at the same time as* it corrects the underlying mechanisms of these symptoms.

How quickly will I feel the result?

One of the best things about the acupuncture treatment of breast disease is that its effects can be immediate. Since the symptoms of breast disease often have to do with stuck qi, as soon as the qi is made to flow, the symptoms begin to disappear and one will feel relief during the treatment itself.

Secondarily, because irritability and nervous tension are also mostly due to liver depression qi stagnation, many women with these adjunctive symptoms will feel immediate relief while still on the table. Typically, one will feel a pronounced tranquility and relaxation within 5-10 minutes of the insertion of the needles.

As for long-term preventive care, we find that a course of seven acupuncture treatments every year or several years seem to be very beneficial for women who are concerned about their risk for developing breast cancer. Most of these women have had premenstrual breast distention and pain or fibrocystic breasts, while others have had fibroadenomas. In this case, we palpate a number a points on the chest and upper back connected with the main channels which traverse the breasts. If any of these are sore to palpation, we needle tem very quickly and very shallowly. Patients receive one treatment per week for four weeks, two treatments spaced every other week in the next month, and a final treatment at the end of the third month. This means we give seven treatments in three months. At the end of that time all premenstrual breast distention and pain are eliminated and the woman can go many months before these return, of course depending on her diet and lifestyle.

Ear acupuncture

Acupuncturists believe there is a map of the entire body in the ear and that by stimulating the corresponding points in the ear, one can remedy those areas and functions of the body. Therefore, many acupuncturists will not only needle points on the body at large but also select one or more points on the ear. In terms of breast disease, ear acupuncture at the Breast point may be effective for relieving pain and distention. Needling the point *Shen Men* (Spirit Gate) can have a profound effect on relaxing tension and irritability and improving sleep.

The nice thing about ear acupuncture points is that one can use tiny "press needles" which are shaped like miniature thumbtacks. These are pressed into the points, covered with adhesive tape, and left in place for five to seven days. This method can provide continuous treatment between regularly scheduled office visits. Thus ear acupuncture is a nice way of extending the duration of an acupuncture treatment. In addition, these ear points can also be stimulated with small metal pellets, radish seeds, or tiny magnets, thus getting the benefits of stimulating these points without having to insert actual needles.

Chinese herbal medicine

The standard of care in China for most gynecological complaints, including breast diseases, emphasizes the use of herbal medicinals. Most often, a woman's prescription will be individually prescribed based on her specific pattern discrimination, not just on a disease diagnosis like PMS or premenstrual breast pain. Women may hear that this or that specific herb is good for relieving breast pain or preventing breast disease but then find that taking the herb did not help them at all. That is because each woman with a given breast *disease* may have varying *patterns* which lead to the occurrence of that disease. We have seen in the breakdown of possible patterns of breast disease listed in Chapter 7. Specifc herbal medicinals are often useful for only one or a couple of these patterns. There is no one medicinal which is effective for treating all patterns of breast disease across the board.

Let's take ginseng as an example. If a woman has fibrocystic breasts but none of her symptoms are due to spleen qi vacuity, then ginseng is not going to help that particular woman. In fact, if her pattern is liver depression transforming into heat or ascendant hyperactivity of liver yang, the woman may very well find herself having more symptoms if she takes enough ginseng long enough. Since this woman's qi is depressed, adding more qi to what is already not flowing freely only adds to this depression which, under pressure, transforms into heat and vents itself upward. On the other hand, if a woman with fibrocystic breast disease does display signs and symptoms of spleen qi vacuity, then the right amount of ginseng is "just what the doctor ordered."

In addition, because most women's breast disorders are a combination of different Chinese patterns and disease mechanisms, professional Chinese medicine never treats women with herbal "singles." In herbalism, singles mean the prescription of a single herb all by itself. Chinese herbal medicine is based on rebalancing patterns, and patterns in real-life patients almost always have more than a single element. Therefore, Chinese doctors almost always prescribe herbs in multi-ingredient formulas. Such formulas may have anywhere from six to 18 or more ingredients. When a Chinese doctor reads a prescription by another Chinese doctor, they can tell you not only what the patient's pattern discrimination is but also their probable signs and symptoms. In other words, the Chinese doctor does not just combine several medicinals which are all reputed to be "good for

123

the breasts," they carefully craft a formula whose ingredients are meant to rebalance every aspect of the patient's body–mind.

Getting your own individualized prescription

Since, in China, it takes not less than four years of full-time college education to learn how to do a professional Chinese pattern discrimination and then write an herbal formula based on that pattern discrimination, most laypeople cannot realistically write their own Chinese herbal prescriptions. It should also be remembered that Chinese herbs are not effective and safe because they are either Chinese or herbal. In fact, approximately 20% of the common Chinese materia medica did not originate in Chinese, and not all Chinese herbs are completely safe. *They are only safe when prescribed according to a correct pattern discrimination, in the right dose, and for the right amount of time.* After all, if an herb is strong enough to heal an imbalance, it is also strong enough to create an imbalance if overdosed or misprescribed.

Therefore, we strongly recommend women who wish to experience the many benefits of Chinese herbal medicine to see a qualified professional practitioner who can do a professional pattern discrimination and write you an individualized prescription. Towards the end of this book, we will give readers suggestions on how to find a qualified professional Chinese medical practitioner near you.

Experimenting with Chinese patent medicines

In reality, qualified professional practitioners of Chinese medicine are not yet found in every North American community. In addition, some women may want to try to heal their symptoms as much on their own as possible. More and more health food stores are stocking a variety of ready-made Chinese formulas in pill and powder form. These ready-made, over the counter Chinese medi-cines are often referred to as Chinese patent

medicines. Although my best recommendation is for wo
seek Chinese herbal treatment from professional practitioners,
below are some suggestions of how one might experiment with
Chinese patent medicines to treat their breast disorders.

In Chapter 7, I have given the signs and symptoms of the key or
basic patterns associated with most women's breast disease. If a
woman can identify her main pattern from this chapter, then
there are some Chinese patent remedies that she might consider
trying.

Xiao Yao Wan (also spelled *Hsiao Yao Wan*)

Xiao Yao Wan is one of the most common Chinese herbal
formulas prescribed to women suffering from PMS and related
diseases. Its Chinese name has been translated as Free & Easy
Pills, Rambling Pills, Relaxed Wanderer Pills, and several other
versions of this same idea of promoting a freer and smoother,
more relaxed flow. As a patent medicine, this formula comes as
pills, and there are both Chinese-made and American-made
versions of this formula available over the counter in the North
American marketplace.[45]

The ingredients in this formula are:

Radix Bupleuri (*Chai Hu*)
Radix Angelicae Sinensis (*Dang Gui*)
Radix Albus Paeoniae Lactiflorae (*Bai Shao*)
Rhizoma Atractylodis Macrocephalae (*Bai Zhu*)
Sclerotium Poriae Cocos (*Fu Ling*)
mix-fried Radx Glycyrrhizae (*Gan Cao*)
Herba Menthae Haplocalycis (*Bo He*)
uncooked Rhizoma Zingiberis (*Sheng Jiang*)

---

[45] When marketed as a dried, powdered extract, this formula is sold under the
name of Bupleurum & Tang-kuei Formula.

125

This formula treats the pattern of liver depression qi stagnation complicated by blood vacuity and spleen weakness with possible dampness as well. Bupleurum courses the liver and rectifies the qi. It is aided in this by Herba Menthae Haplocalycis or Peppermint. Dang Gui and Radix Albus Paeoniae Lactilforae or White Peony nourish the blood and soften and harmonize the liver. Rhizoma Atractylodis Macrocephalae or Atractylodes and Sclerotium Poriae Cocos or Poria fortify the spleen and eliminate dampness. Mix-fried Licorice aid these two in fortifying the spleen and supplementing the liver, while uncooked Ginger aids in both promoting and regulating the qi flow and eliminating dampness.

When breast disorders present with the signs and symptoms of liver depression and spleen vacuity, one can try taking this formula as soon as any symptoms appear and continue taking this formula through the first day of menstruation. However, after taking these pills at the dose recommended on the packaging, if one notices any side effects, then stop immediately and seek a professional consultation. Such side effects from this formula might include nervousness, irritability, a dry mouth and increased thirst, and red, dry eyes. Such side effects show that this formula, at least with modification, is not right for you. Although it may be doing you some good, it is also causing some harm. Remember, Chinese medicine is meant to cure without side effects, and as long as the prescription matches one's pattern there will not be any.

Dan Zhi Xiao Yao Wan

Dan Zhi Xiao Yao Wan or Moutan & Gardenia Rambling Pills is a modification of the above formula which also comes as a patent medicine in the form of pills.[46] It is meant to treat the pattern of liver depression transforming into heat with spleen vacuity and

---

[46] When marketed as a dried, powdered extract, this formula is called Bupleurum & Peony Formula.

possible blood vacuity and/or dampness. The ingredients in this formula are the same as above except that two other herbs are added:

Cortex Radicis Moutan (*Dan Pi*)
Fructus Gardeniae Jasminoidis (*Shan Zhi Zi*)

These two ingedients clear heat and resolve depression. In addition, Cortex Radicis Moutan or Moutan quickens the blood and dispels stasis and is good at clearing heat specifically from the blood. Some Chinese doctors say to take out uncooked Ginger and Mint, while others leave these two ingredients in.

Basically, the signs and symptoms of the pattern for which this formula is designed are the same as those for *Xiao Yao San* above plus signs and symptoms of depressive heat. These might include a reddish tongue with slightly yellow fur, a bowstring and rapid pulse, a bitter taste in the mouth, and increased irritability.

Shu Gan Wan (also spelled *Shu Kan Wan*)

Shu Gan Wan means Soothe the Liver Pills.[47] This Chinese patent medicine is made up almost entirely of liver-coursing and qi-rectifying medicinals. Unlike *Xiao Yao Wan* above, it does not nourish the blood or supplement the spleen. Its ingredients are:

Fructus Meliae Toosendan (*Chuan Lian Zi*)
Rhizoma Curcumae Longae (*Jiang Huang*)
Lignum Aquilariae Agallochae (*Chen Xiang*)
Rhizoma Corydalis Yanhusuo (*Yan Hu Suo*)
Radix Auklandiae Lappae (*Mu Xiang*)
Semen Alpiniae Katsumadai (*Dou Kou*)
Radix Albus Paeoniae Lactiflorae (*Bai Shao*)

---

[47] This formula does not come as a standard dried, powdered formula. However, various companies making such powdered formulas can make it as a special order.

Sclerotium Poriae Cocos (*Fu Ling*)
Fructus Citri Aurantii (*Zhi Ke*)
Pericarpium Citri Reticulatae (*Chen Pi*)
Fructus Amomi (*Sha Ren*)
Cortex Magnoliae Officinalis (*Hou Po*)

This formula can be taken by itself when a woman's symptoms consist of breast and possibly abdominal distention and cramping due to liver depression qi stagnation alone. However, one can also take these pills along with *Xiao Yao Wan* if there is liver depression and spleen and/or blood vacuity with more pronounced breast and/or abdominal distention and menstrual cramps. If taking these pills causes feelings of dryness or heat internally or if they make one even more vexed and irritable, either their dosage should be reduced or they should be stopped.

Xiang Sha Liu Jun Wan

The name of these pills translates as Auklandia & Amomum Six Gentlemen Pills.[48] Sometimes they are referred to as Aplotaxis-Amomum Pills. This formula treats the pattern of pronounced spleen vacuity with elements of dampness and a little qi stagnation. Since the overwhelming majority of women's breast disease includes liver depression qi stagnation, these pills can be taken along with *Xiao Yao Wan* in those cases where spleen vacuity is more severe. These pills are especially good for treating poor appetite, nausea, abdominal bloating after meals, and loose stools due to spleen vacuity and dampness. Their ingredients include:

Radix Codonopsitis Pilosulae (*Dang Shen*)
Rhizoma Atractylodis Macrocephalae (*Bai Zhu*)
Sclerotium Poriae Cocos (*Fu Ling*)
Rhizoma Pinelliae Ternatae (*Ban Xia*)
mix-fried Radix Glycyrrhizae (*Gan Cao*)

---

[48] When sold as a dried, powdered extract, this formula is called Saussurea & Cardamon Combination.

Pericarpium Citri Reticulatae (*Chen Pi*)
Radix Auklandiae Lappae (*Mu Xiang*)
Fructus Amomi (*Sha Ren*)

One should not take these pills, however, if there is burning around the anus with bowel movements or there is diarrhea with dark colored, foul-smelling, explosive stools.

Bu Zhong Yi Qi Wan

Bu Zhong Yi Qi Wan means Supplement the Center & Boost the Qi Pills.[49] This formula treats the pattern of central qi vacuity or central qi fall. The central qi is another name for the spleen and stomach qi. This formula is especially good for treating spleen vacuity weakness manifesting not so much as digestive complaints and diarrhea but as more pronounced fatigue and orthostatic hypotension. Orthostatic hypotension means dizziness on standing up. The ingredients in this formula are:

Radix Astaragli Membranacei (*Huang Qi*)
Radix Codonopsitis Pilosulae (*Dang Shen*)
Rhizoma Atractylodis Macrocephalae (*Bai Zhu*)
mix-fried Radix Glycyrrhizae (*Gan Cao*)
Radix Angelicae Sinensis (*Dang Gui*)
Radix Bupleuri (*Chai Hu*)
Rhizoma Cimicifugae (*Sheng Ma*)
Pericarpium Citri Reticulatae (*Chen Pi*)
Fructus Zizyphi Jujubae (*Da Zao*)
uncooked Rhizoma Zingiberis (*Sheng Jiang*)

This is acutally a very sophisticated formula and it has a very wide range or application. Because it includes Bupleurum and Dang Gui, it courses the liver and rectifies the qi as well as nourishes the blood and softens the liver. It can be added to *Xiao*

---

[49] When sold as a dried, powdered extract, this formula is called Ginseng & Astragalus Combination.

Yao Wan when spleen vacuity causing fatigue is more pronounced. Since spleen vacuity typically does become more pronounced after the age of 35, these pills are often the guiding prescription or are combined with other formulas.

Ba Zhen Wan

Ba Zhen Wan literally means Eight Pearls Pills.[50] However, these are also often marketed under the name Women's Precious Pills. They are called "eight pearls" because they include four ingredients which supplement the qi and four ingredients which nourish the blood. These pills can be combined with *Xiao Yao Wan* when there is liver depression complicated by more serious spleen qi and liver blood vacuity. Their ingredients are:

Radix Codonopsitis Pilosulae (*Dang Shen*)
Rhizoma Atractylodis Macrocephalae (*Bai Zhu*)
Sclerotium Poriae Cocos (*Fu Ling*)
mix-fried Radix Glycyrrhizae (*Gan Cao*)
Radix Angelicae Sinensis (*Dang Gui*)
Radix Albus Paeoniae Lactiflorae (*Bai Shao*)
cooked Radix Rehmanniae (*Shu Di*)
Radix Ligustici Wallichii (*Chuan Xiong*)

Shi Quan Da Bu Wan

The name of these pills translates as Ten (Ingredients) Completely & Greatly Supplementing Pills.[51] Their ingredients are the same as *Ba Zhen Wan* above plus:

Cortex Cinnamomi Cassiae (*Rou Gui*)
Radix Astragali Membranacei (*Huang Qi*)

---

[50] When sold as a dried, powdered extract, this formula is called Tang-kuei & Ginseng Eight Combination.

[51] When sold as a dried, powdered extract, this formula is called Ginseng & Tang-kuei Ten Combination.

Basically they are the same formula. Some Chinese doctors feel that these extra two ingredients help the body generate new qi and blood more rapidly. Therefore, it can be added to *Xiao Yao Wan* for the same reasons as *Ba Zhen Wan*. However, because Cortex Cinnamomi Cassiae or cinnamon bark is hot, it should not be used if there is depressive heat. In other words, one would not usually combine these pills with *Dan Zhi Xiao Yao Wan*.

Tabellae *Suan Zao Ren Tang*

This is a tableted version of the formula, *Suan Zao Ren Tang* (Zizyphus Seed Decoction).[52] It treats insomnia and mental unrest due to liver blood vacuity. It can, therefore, be combined with *Xiao Yao Wan* when liver blood vacuity is more severe and manifests primarily as insomnia. Its ingredients are:

Semen Zizyphi Spinosae (*Suan Zao Ren*)
Sclerotium Poriae Cocos (*Fu Ling*)
Radix Ligustici Wallichii (*Chuan Xiong*)
Rhizoma Anemarrhenae Aspheloidis (*Zhi Mu*)
mix-fried Radix Glycyrrhizae (*Gan Cao*)

Gui Pi Wan (also spelled *Kuei Pi Wan*)

Gui means to return or restore, *pi* means the spleen, and *wan* means pills. Therefore, the name of these pills means Restore the Spleen Pills.[53] However, these pills not only supplement the spleen qi but also nourish heart blood and calm the heart spirit. They are the textbook guiding formula for the pattern of heart-spleen dual vacuity. In this case, there are symptoms of spleen qi vacuity, such as fatigue, poor appetite, and cold hands and feet plus symptoms of heart blood vacuity, such as a pale tongue,

---

[52] When sold as a dried, powdered extract, this formula is called Zizyphus Combination.

[53] When sold as a dried, powdered extract, this formula is called Ginseng & Longan Combination.

heart palpitations, and insomnia. This formula is also the standard one for treating heavy or abnormal bleeding due to the spleen not containing and restraining the blood within its vessels. Therefore, this patent medicine can be combined with *Xiao Yao San* when there is liver depression qi stagnation complicated by heart blood and spleen qi vacuity. Its ingredients are:

Radix Astragali Membranacei (*Huang Qi*)
Radix Codonopsitis Pilosulae (*Dang Shen*)
Rhizoma Atractylodis Macrocephalae (*Bai Zhu*)
Sclerotium Parardicis Poriae Cocos (*Fu Shen*)
mix-fried Radix Glycyrrhizae (*Gan Cao*)
Radix Angelicae Sinensis (*Dang Gui*)
Semen Zizyphi Spinosae (*Suan Zao Ren*)
Arillus Euphoriae Longanae (*Long Yan Rou*)
Radix Polygalae Tenuifoliae (*Yuan Zhi*)
Radix Auklandiae Lappae (*Mu Xiang*)

Er Chen Wan

Er Chen Wan means Two Aged (Ingredients) Pills.[54] This is because two of its main ingredients are aged before using. This formula is used to transform phlegm and eliminate dampness. It can be added to *Xiao Yao Wan* if there is liver depression with spleen vacuity and more pronounced phlegm and dampness. Its ingredients include:

Rhizoma Pinelliae Ternatae (*Ban Xia*)
Sclerotium Poriae Cocos (*Fu Ling*)
mix-fried Radix Glycyrrhizae (*Gan Cao*)
Pericarpium Citri Reticulatae (*Chen Pi*)
uncooked Rhizoma Zingiberis (*Sheng Jiang*)

---

[54] When sold as a dried, powdered extract, this formula is called Citrus & Pinellia Combination.

Ge Jie Da Bu Wan

Gecko Greatly Supplementing Pills supplement the qi, blood, yin, and yang. It is usually used to treat low back and lower limb pain associated with kidney vacuity in turn due to aging. Because most women develop not only spleen vacuity but also kidney yin and yang vacuity as they move towards menopause in their late 40s, this formula can be combined with *Xiao Yao Wan* when there is liver depression, spleen and kidney yang vacuity, and blood and yin vacuity as well. The ingredients in this Chinese patent medicine include:

Gecko (*Ge Jie*)
Radix Astragali Membranacei (*Huang Qi*)
Radix Codonopsitis Pilosulae (*Dang Shen*)
Fructus Lycii Chinensis (*Gou Qi Zi*)
Radix Angelicae Sinensis (*Dang Gui*)
cooked Radix Rehmanniae (*Shu Di*)
Fructus Ligustri Lucidi (*Nu Zhen Zi*)
Rhizoma Polygonati (*Huang Jing*)
Rhizoma Atractylodis Macrocephalae (*Bai Zhu*)
Sclerotium Poriae Cocos (*Fu Ling*)
Radix Dioscoreae Oppositae (*Shan Yao*)
Radix Glycyrrhizae (*Gan Cao*)
Cortex Eucommiae Ulmoidis (*Du Zhong*)
Radix Dipsaci (*Xu Duan*)
Rhizoma Cibotii Barmetsis (*Gou Ji*)
Radix Morindae Officinalis (*Ba Ji Tian*)
Rhizoma Drynariae (*Gu Sui Bu*)
Fructus Chaenomelis Lagenariae (*Mu Gua*)

The above Chinese patent medicines only give a suggestion of how one or several over the counter Chinese ready-made preparations may be used to treat breast diseases accompanied by a wide variety of other symptoms. As professional practitioners ourselves who know how hard it is to practice Chinese medicine correctly even after years of training, we prefer to see women receive a professional diagnosis and an individually tailored prescription. However, as long as one is careful to try to match up their pattern with the right formula and not to exceed the recommended dosage, one can try treating their own symptoms with one or more of these remedies. If it works, great! These patent medicines are usually quite cheap. If this approach doesn't work after a few menstrual cycles or if there are *any side effects*, one should stop and see a professional practitioner.

In general, you can tell if any medication and treatment are good for you by checking the following six guideposts.

1. Digestion
2. Elimination
3. Energy level

4. Mood
5. Appetite
6. Sleep

If a medication, be it modern Western or traditional Chinese, gets rid of your symptoms and all six of these basic areas of human health improve or are fine to begin with, then that medicine or treatment is probably OK. However, even if a treatment or medication takes away your major complaint, if it causes deterioration in one of these six basic parameters, then that treatment or medication is probably not OK and is certainly not OK for long–term use. When medicines and treatments, even so-called natural, herbal medications, are prescribed based on a person's pattern of disharmony, then there is healing without side effects. According to Chinese medicine, this is the only kind of true healing.

Chinese Medical Research on Breast Disease

Considerable research has been done in the People's Republic of China on the effects of acupuncture and Chinese herbal medicine on a variety of breast diseases. Usually, this research is in the form of a clinical audit. That means that a group of patients with the same diseases, patterns, or major complaints are given the same treatment for a certain period of time. After this time, the patients are counted to see how many were cured, how many got a marked effect, how many got some effect, and how many got no effect. This kind of "outcome-based research" has, up until only very recently, not been considered credible in the West where, for the last 30 years or so, the double-blind, placebo-controlled comparison study has been considered the "gold standard." However, such double-blind, placebo-controlled comparison studies are impossible to design in Chinese medicine and do not, in any case, measure effectiveness in a real-life situation.

Clinical audits, on the other hand, do measure actual clinical satisfaction of real-life patients. Such clinical audits may not exclude the patient's trust and belief in the therapist or the therapy as an important component in the result. However, real-life is not as neat and discreet as a controlled laboratory experiment. If the majority of patients are satisfied with the results of a particular treatment and there are no adverse side effects to that treatment, then that is good enough for the Chinese doctor, and, in my experience, that is also good enough for the vast majority of my patients.

Below are abbreviated translations of several recent research articles published in Chinese medical journals on the treatment of premenstrual breast distention and pain and fibrocystic disease. Many women with premenstrual breast distention and pain also have fibrocystic breasts, and typically, fibrocystic breasts do get worse during the premenstruum. These research articles exemplify how Chinese medicine treats one of the most common premenstrual complaints. We think that most women reading these statistics would think that Chinese medicine was worth a try.

"The Pattern Discrimination Treatment of 90 Cases of Menstrual Movement Breast Distention" by Wang Fa-chang & Wang Qu-an, *Shan Dong Zhong Yi Za Zhi (The Shandong Journal of Chinese Medicine)*, #5, 1993, p. 24-25

Menstrual movement, *i.e.*, premenstrual, breast distention and pain is one of the most commonly seen complaints in gynecology departments. The authors of this clinical audit have treated 90 cases of this condition based on pattern discrimination. Of these 90 women, 4 were between 16-20 years old, 11 between 21-25, 20 between 26-30, 21 between 31-35, 20 between 36-40, 5 between 41-45, 7 between 46-50, and 2 cases were more than 50 years old. The course of these women's disease was from one half year to 20 years.

1. Simultaneous liver depression with damp heat pattern

The main symptoms of this pattern are premenstrual chest oppression, heart vexation and easy anger, breast distention and pain, a dry mouth, vexatious heat of the chest and epigastrium, lower abdominal aching and pain, possible vaginal itching or excessive, yellow-colored vaginal discharge, a bowstring, rapid pulse, and red tongue with thin, yellow fur. The treatment principles were to course the liver and resolve depression, clear heat and disinhibit dampness. The formula consisted of a combination of *Dan Zhi Xiao Yao San* (Moutan & Gardenia

136

Rambling Powder), *Yi Huang Tang* (Change Yellow [Discharge] Decoction), and *San Miao San* (Three Wonders Powder) plus Rhizoma Cyperi Rotundi (*Xiang Fu*).

2. Simultaneous liver depression with blood stasis pattern

The main symptoms of this pattern are premenstrual heart vexation and easy anger, breast distention and pain, occasional nodulation, lower abdominal distention and pain disliking pressure, possible scanty menstruation which does not come smoothly, a dark, purplish menstruate containing clots, a bowstring, slippery pulse, and a purplish, dark tongue with static spots or patches and thin, white fur. The treatment principles were to course the liver and resolve depression, quicken the blood, transform stasis, and stop pain. The formula consisted of *Dan Zhi Xiao Yao San* (Moutan & Gardenia Rambling Powder) combined with *Tao Hong Si Wu Tang* (Persica & Carthamus Four Materials Decoction) plus Pericarpium Citri Reticulatae Viride (*Qing Pi*), Rhizoma Corydalis Yanhusuo (*Yan Hu Suo*), and Tuber Curcumae (*Yu Jin*).

3. Simultaneous liver depression with heart/spleen dual vacuity pattern

The main symptoms of this pattern are premenstrual chest oppression, heart vexation and chaotic thoughts, mild, insidious breast pain or small sensations of distention, heart palpitations, dizziness, loss of sleep, profuse dreaming, lack of strength of the entire body, lassitude of the spirit, diminished appetite, excessive, pasty white vaginal discharge, a bowstring, fine pulse, and a pale tongue with teeth marks on its border and thin, white fur. The treatment principles were to course the liver and resolve depression, fortify the spleen and harmonize the stomach, nourish the heart and quiet the spirit. The formula consisted of *Dan Shen Gui Pi Tang* (Salvia Restore the Spleen Decoction) plus Rhizoma Cyperi Rotundi (*Xiang Fu*) and Tuber Curcumae (*Yu Jin*).

137

4. Liver/kidney insufficiency pattern

The main symptoms of this pattern are premenstrual chest oppression, heart vexation and chaotic thoughts, mild, insidious breast pain, dizziness, tinnitus, low back pain, weakness of the extremities, lack of strength, a deep, bowstring pulse, and a pale tongue with scanty fur. The treatment principles were to course the liver and fortify the spleen, supplement and boost the liver and kidneys. The formula consisted of *Dan Zhi Xiao Yao San* (Moutan & Gardenia Rambling Powder) plus Cortex Eucommiae Ulmoidis (*Du Zhong*), Radix Dipsaci (*Chuan Xu Duan*), Ramulus Loranthi Seu Visci (*Sang Ji Sheng*), Cornu Degelatinum Cervi (*Lu Jiao Shuang*), Fructus Corni Officinalis (*Shan Zhu Yu*), and Semen Cuscutae (*Tu Si Zi*).

5. Simultaneous liver depression with *chong* and *ren* vacuity cold pattern

The main symptoms of this pattern are premenstrual heart vexation and chaotic thoughts, lassitude of the spirit, breast distention and pain, insidious lower abdominal pain with a cool sensation, a fine, slow pulse, and a pale tongue with thin, white fur. The treatment principles were to course the liver and resolve depression, cherish the palace (*i.e.*, uterus) and scatter cold. The formula consisted of *Dan Zhi Xiao Yao San* (Moutan & Gardenia Rambling Powder) plus Radix Linderae Strychnifoliae (*Wu Yao*), Rhizoma Cyperi Rotundi (*Xiang Fu*), stir-fried Fructus Foeniculi Vulgaris (*Xiao Hui Xiang*), and stir-fried Folium Artemisiae Argyii (*Ai Ye*).

One course of treatment consisted of three bags of the above formula administered during the woman's premenstruum, one bag being brewed as a "tea" and taken each day. Complete cure was defined as disappearance of such symptoms as premenstrual chest oppression, heart vexation and chaotic thoughts, breast distention and pain, etc. with reduction or disappearance of nodulations and lumps in the breasts within three courses of treatment, *i.e.*, three menstrual cycles. Marked improvement consisted of reduction in such symptoms as premenstrual chest oppression, heart vexation and chaotic thoughts, breast distention and pain, etc. within three courses of treatment. Fair improvement consisted of reduction in the same sorts of symptoms as above in three courses of treatment but recurrence or worsening of these symptoms due to emotional stress. Of the 90 women treated in this study, 57 were cured, 23 were markedly improved, eight experienced fair improvement, and two got no result. Thus the total amelioration rate using this protocol was 97.8%.

"The Treatment of 24 Cases of Fibrocystic Breasts with *Ru Kuai Xiao Tang Jia Wei* (Breast Lump Dispersing Decoction with Added Flavors" by Hou Jian, *Shan Dong Zhong Yi Za Zhi (The Shandong Journal of Chinese Medicine)*, #5, 1993, p. 33

This clinical audit reports on the treatment of 24 cases of fibrocystic breast disease with *Ru Kuai Xiao Tang Jia Wei* from 1989-1991. The age of the women in this study ranged from 23-50 years old, with six cases being between 23-30, 15 between 31-40, and three between 41-50 years of age. Thirteen cases had suffered from this condition for six months or less, five cases from seven months to one year, and six cases for over one year. All these women were married. Treatment used a basic formula which was modified based on pattern discrimination.

1. Liver qi depression & stagnation pattern (13 cases)

The signs and symptoms of this pattern include breast distention and pain which occurred either before the period or got worse with the approach of the period, pain and distention reaching the chest and lateral costal regions, palpable fibrotic tissue and lumps within the breasts but without clearly demarcated borders, lumps may be changeable (*i.e.*, come and go, grow and shrink with the menstrual cycle), lack of ease in emotional affairs, sighing, chest oppression, a darkish pale tongue with thin, white fur, and a bowstring, fine pulse.

2. Phlegm congelation, blood stasis pattern (7 cases)

The signs and symptoms of this pattern include dull breast pain and numbness. However, in prolonged cases, there is piercing pain. In addition there are nodular lumps which do not adhere to the underside of the skin and which are pliable and not hard. Typically, there is physical fatigue, nausea, vomiting of phlegmy saliva, a gloomy (*i.e.*, darkish) tongue with glossy, slimy fur, and a slippery or choppy pulse.

3. *Chong* & *ren* loss of regulation pattern (4 cases)

The signs and symptoms of this pattern include breast heaviness and pain, many breast lumps spread all over the place occurring before, with, or after menstruation, emotional tension, agitation and easy anger, low back soreness, lack of strength, a pale tongue with white fur, and a soggy or vacuous pulse. This pattern mostly occurs in older women.

Ru Kuai Xiao Tang (the basic formula used in this protocol) consisted of: Fructus Trichosanthis Kirlowii (*Gua Lou*), 15g, uncooked Concha Ostreae (*Mu Li*), 15g, Spica Prunellae Vulgaris (*Xia Gu Cao*), 15g, Thallus Algae (*Kun Bu*), 15g, Herba Sargassii (*Hai Zao*), 15g, Radix Salviae Miltiorrhizae (*Dan Shen*), 15g, Radix Bupleuri (*Chai Hu*), 9g, Tuber Asparagi Cochinensis (*Tian Men Dong*), 9g, Rhizoma Sparganii (*San Leng*), 9g, Rhizoma Curcumae Zedoariae (*E Zhu*), 9g, Folium Citri (*Ju Ye*), 9g, Semen Citri (*Ju He*), 9g, and Rhizoma Pinelliae Ternatae (*Ban Xia*), 9g. These were decocted in water and administered in two divided doses, one bag per day. Treatment was commenced 15 days before the onset of the period, with 12 days equalling one course of treatment. Administration of these medicinals was discontinued during the period itself.

If the pattern was liver qi depression & stagnation, Pericarpium Citri Reticulatae Viride (*Qing Pi*) and Rhizoma Cyperi Rotundi (*Xiang Fu*), 9g @, were added to move the qi and scatter depression. If the pattern was phlegm congelation and blood stasis, the amounts of Concha Ostreae, Thallus Algae, and Radix Salviae Miltiorrhizae were increased up to 30g @ to soften the hard and dispel stasis. If the pattern was *chong* and *ren* loss of regulation, Radix Morindae Officinalis (*Ba Ji Tian*), Cornu Degelatinum Cervi (*Lu Jiao Shuang*), and Retinervus Luffae Cyclindricae (*Si Gua Luo*) were added to secure the kidneys, rectify the *chong*, and free the flow of the network vessels in the breasts.

Complete cure consisted of disappearance of the breast lumps, complete reduction in the aching and pain, and no recurrence on follow-up a half year later. Some improvement was defined as reduction in the size of the lumps and diminishment in the pain and soreness. No results meant that there was no change in either the lumps or the pain. Based on these criteria, in one course of treatment, six women were cured and four got some improvement. In two courses of treatment, three more women were cured and two more got some improvement. In three courses of treatment, three additional women were cured and one more got some improvement. And in four courses of treatment, one more was cured, two more improved, and two got no result. Therefore, the total number of cases cured was 13. The total number of cases improved was nine. And only two women experienced no result. Thus the total amelioration rate was 91.7%.

The author of this article quotes the *Wai Ke Zheng Zong (The True Lineage of External Medicine)* in explaining how this condition comes about:

> Breast aggregation (the traditional Chinese medical name for fibrocystic breasts and breast lumps) consists of nodulations within the breast, their form being like that of an egg. They may be heavy and painful or there may be no pain. The skin (above them) is not changed. These kernels' growth and decline may follow the (growth and decline of) joy and anger. They are mostly due to worry and anxiety damaging the spleen and irritation and anger damaging the liver with depression binding becoming (nodulation).

"50 Cases Treated for Premenstrual Breast Distention & Pain with *Jie Yu Huo Xue Tang* (Resolve Depression & Quicken the Blood Decoction)" by Gu Si-yun, *Shan Dong Zhong Yi Za Zhi (The Shandong Journal of Chinese Medicine)*, # 6, 1992, p. 27-28

The author of this study begins by saying that premenstrual breast distention is primarily due to liver depression and qi stagnation with subsequent loss of harmony and downbearing of the stomach. Since the breasts are primarily circulated by the liver and stomach channels, qi depression and stagnation affecting these two organs make it difficult for the qi to drain from these channels as they should. Fifty women suffering from premenstrual breast distention and pain were, therefore, treated with the following formula: Radix Bupleuri (*Chai Hu*), 12g, Rhizoma Cyperi Rotundi (*Xiang Fu*), 15g, Radix Ligustici Wallichii (*Chuan Xiong*), 12g, Fructus Citri Aurantii (*Zhi Ke*), 9g, Radix Rubrus Paeoniae Lactiflorae (*Chi Shao*), 12g, Semen Pruni Persicae (*Tao Ren*), 10g, Flos Carthami Tinctorii (*Hong Hua*), 9g, Pericarpium Citri Reticulatae Viride (*Qing Pi*), 10g, Folium Citri (*Ju Ye*), 10g, Fructus Trichosanthis Kirlowii (*Gua Lou*), 15g, Radix Glycyrrhizae (*Gan Cao*), 6g, Radix Salviae Miltiorrhizae (*Dan Shen*), 15g, Tuber Curcumae (*Yu Jin*), 12g, Radix Dioscoreae Oppositae (*Shan Yao*), 12g.

If patients suffered from spleen vacuity, Radix Codonopsitis Pilosulae (*Dang Shen*), Radix Astragali Membranacei (*Huang Qi*), Rhizoma Atractylodis (*Cang Zhu*), Rhizoma Atractylodis Macrocephalae (*Bai Zhu*), and Fructus Amomi (*Sha Ren*) were added. If patients suffered from blood vacuity, Radix Angelicae Sinensis (*Dang Gui*), cooked Radix Rehmanniae (*Shu Di*), and Radix Albus Paeoniae Lactiflorae (*Bai Shao*) were added. If patients suffered from kidney yang vacuity, Cortex Eucommiae Ulmoidis (*Du Zhong*), Semen Cuscutae (*Tu Si Zi*), Radix Dipsaci (*Xu Duan*), and Herba Epimedii (*Yin Yang Huo*) were added. If patients suffered from kidney yin vacuity, Rhizoma Anemarrhenae Aspheloidis (*Zhi Mu*), uncooked Radix Rehmanniae (*Sheng Di*), Fructus Corni Officinalis (*Shan Zhu Yu*), and Herba Ecliptae Prostratae (*Han Lian Cao*) were added. For liver fire

142

invading the stomach, Fructus Gardeniae Jasminoidis (*Zhi Zi*), Cortex Radicis Moutan (*Dan Pi*), and Pericarpium Citri Reticulatae (*Chen Pi*) were added. For ascendant hyperactivity of liver yang, Ramulus Uncariae Cum Uncis (*Gou Teng*), Concha Margaritiferae (*Zhen Zhu Mu*), Radix Gentianae Scabrae (*Long Dan Cao*), and Flos Chrysanthemi Morifolii (*Ju Hua*) were added. For yin vacuity and yang hyperactivity, Concha Ostreae (*Mu Li*), Gelatinum Corii Asini (*E Jiao*), Tuber Ophiopogonis Japonici (*Mai Dong*), and uncooked Radix Rehmanniae (*Sheng Di*) were added. If there was blood stasis and phlegm congelation, Radix Angelicae Sinensis (*Dang Gui*), Squama Manitis Pentadactylis (*Chuan Shan Jia*), Semen Vaccariae Segetalis (*Wang Bu Liu Xing*), and Rhizoma Sparganii (*San Leng*) were added. These ingredients were decocted in water and one packet of the above herbal medicinals were given per day.

Of the women treated in this study, the oldest was 35 and the youngest was 15 years of age. Twenty women were between the ages of 15 and 20. Eighteen were between the ages of 21 and 30, and 12 were 31 or older. The duration of their disease had lasted from a minimum of six months to a maximum of 10 years, with the average being three years. The above treatment was given for three whole months. At the end of that time, 44 cases or 88% experienced complete cure. Another five cases or 10% experienced some improvement. While only a single case or 2% failed to experience any improvement. Thus the total amelioration rate of the patients participating in this study was 98%.

"The Treatment of 128 Cases of Fibrocystic Breasts" by Mi Yang, *Hu Nan Zhong Yi Za Zhi (The Hunan Journal of Chinese Medicine)*, #1, 1993, p. 47

This clinical audit describes the treatment of 128 cases of fibrocystic breast disease using a formula called *Shen Xiao Gua Lou San*. Sixty-eight cases involved women between the ages of 22-30, 46 cases, 31-40, and 14 cases, 41-55 years of age.

The formula used was *Shen Xiao Gua Lou San* (Magically Dispersing Trichosanthes Powder): Fructus Trichosanthis Kirlowii (*Quan Gua Lou*), 15g, processed Resina Olibani (*Ru Xiang*) and processed Resina Myrrhae (*Mo Yao*), 10g @, Radix Angelicae Sinensis (*Dang Gui*), 12g, and Radix Glycyrrhizae (*Gan Cao*), 6g. These were boiled in 500 ml of water, one packet per day, taken in two divided doses.

If it was possible to feel swelling and lumps within the breast and the emotions were not easy and if there were chest and lateral costal pain and fullness, heart vexation and easy anger, premenstrual breast distention and pain, swelling and lumps which felt achy and painful as if heavy, and pressure caused worsening of the pain, then Radix Bupleuri (*Chai Hu*), Radix Rubrus Paeoniae Lactiflorae (*Chi Shao*), Semen Vaccariae Segetalis (*Wang Bu Liu Xing*), and stir-fried Fructus Citri Aurantii (*Zhi Ke*) were added to this formula. If the breast lumps were stringy or ropy within the breasts or scattered throughout the breasts, if their nature was pliable but tough, menstruation was excessive but pale in color, the four limbs were without strength, and there were dizziness and vertigo, Radix Astragali Membranacei (*Huang Qi*), Radix Codonopsitis Pilosulae (*Dang Shen*), and Fructus Liquidambaris Taiwaniae (*Lu Lu Tong*) were added. If the breasts were swollen and painful and scorching hot, the tongue was red with thin, yellow fur, and the pulse was bowstring and rapid, Flos Lonicerae Japonicae (*Jin Yin Hua*), Fructus Forsythiae Suspensae (*Lian Qiao*), and Herba Taraxaci Mongolici Cum Radice (*Pu Gong Ying*) were added. If the breast lumps were comparatively firm but not hard, if pressure caused aching and pain, and the lumps shifted position when pushed, blast-fried Squama Manitis Pentadactylis (*Chuan Shan Jia*), Spina Gleditschiae Chinensis (*Zao Jiao Ci*), Rhizoma Sparganii (*San Leng*), and Rhizoma Curcumae Zedoariae (*E Zhu*) were added.

Treatment lasted between 30-180 days, with the average being 50 days. Complete cure was defined as disappearance of the lumps. Marked improvement was defined as diminishment of the pain and aching and decrease in the size of the lumps. No result was defined as no diminishment in the pain or aching and no decrease in the size of the lumps. Based on these criteria, 80 cases (62.5%) of the women in this study experienced complete cure; 42 (32.81%) experienced marked improvement; and six cases got no result. Thus the total amelioration rate was 95.31%.

"The Pattern Discrimination Treatment of 100 Cases of Fibro-cystic Breasts" by Fang Jian-ping, *Jiang Su Zhong Yi (Jiangsu Chinese Medicine)*, #2, 1993, p. 14

This research report describes the treatment of 100 cases of fibrocystic breast disease based on treating according to a discrimination of patterns. Four patients were between the ages of 15-20; 25 between 21-30; 54 between 31-40; and there were 17 cases between 41-50 years of age. Ninety were married and 10 were unmarried.

1. Liver depression, qi stagnation pattern (45 cases)

The lumps within these women's breasts were large like date pits or chicken eggs. They also presented with emotional lability, heart vexation, and easy anger. The women's menstruation was not easy and there was premenstrual breast heaviness and discomfort, distention and pain. The tongue fur was thin, white or yellow, and the pulse was bowstring. The therapeutic principles were to course the liver and resolve depression, move the qi and scatter nodulation. The formula used was *Xiao Yao San Jia Jian* (Rambling Powder with Additions & Subtractions): vinegar-fried Radix Bupleuri (*Chai Hu*) and stir-fried Fructus Gardeniae Jasminoidis (*Shan Zhi Zi*), 5g @, Radix Albus Paeoniae Lacti-florae (*Bai Shao*), Sclerotium Poriae Cocos (*Fu Ling*), Radix Angelicae Sinensis (*Dang Gui*), Herba Taraxaci Mongolici Cum Radice (*Pu Gong Ying*), Pericarpium Trichosanthis Kirlowii (*Gua Lou Pi*), Pericarpium Citri Reticulatae Viride (*Qing Pi*), Rhizoma Atractylodis Macrocephalae (*Bai Zhu*), and Semen Citri (*Ju He*), 10g @, roasted Rhizoma Zingiberis (*Wei Jiang*) and Radix

Glycyrrhizae (*Gan Cao*), 3g @, and processed Squama Manitis Pentadactylis (*Chuan Shan Jia*), 6g.

2. Liver depression, qi vacuity pattern (23 cases)

These women's lumps were divided and scattered or blended into the rest of the tissue and were not easily discernable. They were also movable. Their facial color was sallow white and they had dizziness and vertigo, were exhausted and lacked strength. Their menses were excessive but pale in color, and their tongues were pale with thin, white fur. Their pulses were soggy and fine. The therapeutic principles for this presentation were to course the liver and scatter nodulation, boost the qi and nourish the blood. The formula used was *Si Wu Tang Jia Jian* (Four Materials Decoction with Additions & Subtractions): cooked Radix Rehmanniae (*Shu Di*), Radix Angelicae Sinensis (*Dang Gui*), Radix Albus Paeoniae Lactiflorae (*Bai Shao*), Radix Astragali Membranacei (*Huang Qi*), Sclerotium Poriae Cocos (*Fu Ling*), Tuber Curcumae (*Yu Jin*), Herba Taraxaci Mongolici Cum Radice (*Pu Gong Ying*), and Fructus Liquidambaris Taiwaniae (*Lu Lu Tong*), 10g @, Radix Ligustici Wallichii (*Chuan Xiong*) and Cornu Degelatinum Cervi (*Lu Jiao Shuang*), 5g @, vinegar-fried Radix Bupleuri (*Chai Hu*), 3g, processed Squama Manitis Pentadactylis (*Chuan Shan Jia*), 6g.

3. Liver depression, phlegm nodulation pattern (18 cases)

These women's lumps were disciform or lobular in shape. Their chests, lateral costal regions, and epigastriums were oppressed and distended accompanied by dizziness, a slightly bitter taste in the mouth, abnormal appetite, clots within their menstrual flow, possible loose stools, a pale tongue with white, slimy fur, and a slippery pulse. The therapeutic principles in this case were to course the liver and flush phlegm, soften the hard and scatter nodulation. The formula used was *Lou Feng Fang Tang Jia Jian* (Nidus Vespae Decoction with Additions & Subtractions): Nidus Vespae (*Lou Feng Fang*), Bulbus Cremastrae (*Shan Ci Gu*), processed Squama Manitis Pentadactylis (*Chuan Shan Jia*), and

Radix Bupleuri (*Chai Hu*), 6g @, Tuber Curcumae (*Yu Jin*), Pericarpium Citri Reticulatae Viride (*Qing Pi*), Bulbus Fritillariae Thunbergii (*Bei Mu*), Folium Citri (*Ju Ye*), 10g @, processed Rhizoma Cyperi Rotundi (*Xiang Fu*), 12g, and Spica Prunellae Vulgaris (*Xia Gu Cao*), 25g.

4. Qi stagnation, blood stasis pattern (14 cases)

These women's lumps were comparatively firm and like a hard ball in shape. They might also be disciform or lobular. There was aching and pain or pain upon pressure. These lumps had been soft or slippery but had undergone a change. There were clots in these women's menstruate and its color was purplish and dark. Their tongues were purple in color or had purple patches. Their pulses were fine and bowstring. The therapeutic principles in this case were to quicken the blood and dispel stasis, soften the hard and scatter nodulation. The formula used was *Jie Yu Ruan Jian Tang* (Resolve Depression & Soften the Hard Decoction): Radix Angelicae Sinensis (*Dang Gui*), mix-fried Radix Rubrus Paeoniae Lactiflorae (*Chi Shao*), Fructus Tribuli Terrestris (*Bai Ji Li*), Thallus Algae (*Kun Bu*), Herba Sargassii (*Hai Zao*), Cornu Degelatinum Cervi (*Lu Jiao Shuang*), Radix Salviae Miltiorrhizae (*Dan Shen*), and Fructus Crataegi (*Shan Zha*), 10g @, processed Rhizoma Cyperi Rotundi (*Xiang Fu*), processed Squama Manitis Pentadactylis (*Chuan Shan Jia*), and Tuber Curcumae (*Yu Jin*), 6g @, Radix Ligustici Wallichii (*Chuan Xiong*), Radix Bupleuri (*Chai Hu*), Pericarpium Citri Reticulatae Viride (*Qing Pi*), and Bulbus Cremastrae (*Shan Ci Gu*), 5g @, and Herba Taraxaci Mongolici Cum Radice (*Pu Gong Ying*), 12g. The above medicinals were administered in decoction internally. At the same time, externally, *Xiao Yan Gao* (Disperse Inflammation Plaster) plus *Ru Kuai San* (Breast Lump Powder, which is composed of Borneolum, *Bing Pian*, Borax, *Yue Shi*, etc.) were applied above the lumps.

The criteria for success using these protocols were as follows: Complete cure was defined as disappearance of the lumps, disappearance of the breast pain, and discontinuance of the medicinals after three months. Marked improvement was defined

147

as diminishment of the size of the lumps by half and disappearance of the breast pain. Some improvement was defined as diminishment of the size of the lumps by less than half and reduction in the breast pain. No result was defined as no reduction in the size of the breast lumps.

Thirty-seven cases of liver depression, qi stagnation experienced complete cure; six, marked improvement; and two, some improvement. Sixteen cases of liver depression, qi vacuity experienced complete cure; five, marked improvement; and two, some improvement. Eleven cases of qi depression, phlegm nodulation experienced complete cure; five, marked improvement; one, some improvement; and one, no result. And eight cases of qi stagnation, blood stasis experienced complete cure; three, marked improvement; one, some improvement; and two, no result. Therefore, the total number of cures was 72; marked improvement, 19; some improvement, six; and no result, three. Thus the total amelioration rate was 97%.

Finding a Professional Practitioner of Chinese Medicine

Traditional Chinese medicine is one of the fastest growing holistic health care systems in the West today. At the present time, there are 50 colleges in the United States alone which offer 3-4 year training programs in acupuncture, moxibustion, Chinese herbal medicine, and Chinese medical massage. In addition, many of the graduates of these programs have done postgraduate studies at colleges and hospitals in China, Taiwan, Hong Kong, and Japan. Further, a growing number of trained Oriental medical practitioners have immigrated from China, Japan, and Korea to practice acupuncture and Chinese herbal medicine in the West.

Traditional Chinese medicine, including acupuncture, is a discreet and independent health care profession. It is not simply a technique that can easily be added to the array of techniques of some other health care profession. The study of Chinese medicine, acupuncture, and Chinese herbs is as rigorous as is the study of allopathic, chiropractic, naturopathic, or homeopathic medicine. Previous training in any one of these other systems does not automatically confer competence or knowledge in Chinese medicine. In order to get the full benefits and safety of Chinese medicine, one should seek out professionally trained and credentialed practitioners.

In the United States of America, recognition that acupuncture and Chinese medicine are their own independent professions has led to the creation of the National Commission for the Certification of Acupuncture & Oriental Medicine (NCCAOM). This commission has created and administers a national board examination in both acupuncture and Chinese herbal medicine in order to insure minimum levels of professional competence and safety. Those who pass the acupuncture exam append the letters Dipl. Ac. (Diplomate of Acupuncture) after their names, while those who pass the Chinese herbal exam use the letters Dipl. C.H. (Diplomate of Chinese Herbs). I recommend that persons wishing to experience the benefits of acupuncture and Chinese medicine should seek treatment in the U.S. only from those who are NCCAOM certified.

In addition, in the United States, acupuncture is a legal, independent health care profession in more than half the states. A few other states require acupuncturists to work under the supervision of MDs, while in a number of states, acupuncture has yet to receive legal status. In states where acupuncture is licensed and regulated, the names of acupuncture practitioners can be found in the *Yellow Pages* of your local phone book or through contacting your State Department of Health, Board of Medical Examiners, or Department of Regulatory Agencies. In states without licensure, it is doubly important to seek treatment only from NCCAOM diplomates.

When seeking a qualified and knowledgeable practitioner, word of mouth referrals are important. Satisfied patients are the most reliable credential a practitioner can have. It is appropriate to ask the practitioner for references from previous patients treated for the same problem. It is best to work with a practitioner who communicates effectively enough for the patient to feel understood and for the Chinese medical diagnosis and treatment plan to make sense. In all cases, a professional practitioner of Chinese medicine should be able and willing to give a written traditional Chinese diagnosis of the patient's pattern upon request.

For further information regarding the practice of Chinese medicine and acupuncture in the United States and for referrals to local professional associations and practitioners in the United States, prospective patients may contact:

National Commission for the Certification of Acupuncture & Oriental Medicine
P.O. Box 97075
Washington DC 20090-7075
Tel: (202) 232-1404
Fax: (202) 462-6157

The National Acupuncture & Oriental Medicine Alliance
14637 Starr Rd, SE
Olalla, WA 98357
Tel: (206) 851-6895
Fax: (206) 728-4841
E mail: 76143.2061@compuserve.com

The American Association of Oriental Medicine
433 Front St.
Catasauqua, PA 18032-2506
Tel: (610) 433-2448
Fax: (610) 433-1832

Conclusion

According to the tenets of Chinese medical theory, minor breast disorders should not be left untreated, nor are they unavoidable discomforts of womanhood. Even the presence of simple breast tenderness before the period is a symptom of minor imbalance which can and should be corrected or improved.

By treating these simple disorders effectively, a woman can help herself avoid more serious ones in later years. The occurrence of such problems as dysfunctional uterine bleeding, uterine fibroids, debilitating premenstrual syndrome, certain types of infertility, endometriosis, menopausal syndrome, and breast tumors both malignant and benign, are all related to this same group of imbalances and can all be lessened or eliminated by traditional Chinese medicine. By treating any of these, one may also prevent the arisal of serious disorders in all other related parts of their body.

It is our hope that through the insights and wisdom of Chinese medicine presented in this book, the pain and suffering of many women may be lessened or eliminated. For *most* breast diseases, it is certain that Chinese medicine offers a logical, rational description of their nature and progression, and effective therapies for their treatment. More importantly, the treatments for these imbalances put a great deal of power and control directly in the hands of women themselves, which is perhaps the greatest gift we are offering with this publication.

Learning More About Chinese Medicine

For more information on Chinese medicine in general, see:

The Web That Has No Weaver: Understanding Chinese Medicine by Ted Kaptchuk, Congdon & Weed, NY, 1983. This is the best overall introduction to Chinese medicine for the serious lay reader. It has been a standard since it was first published over a dozen years ago and it has yet to be replaced.

Chinese Secrets of Health & Longevity by Bob Flaws, Sound True, Boulder, CO, 1996. This is a six tape audiocassette course introducing Chinese medicine to laypeople. It covers basic Chinese medical theory, Chinese dietary therapy, Chinese herbal medicine, acupuncture, *qi gong, feng shui,* deep relaxation, lifestyle, and more.

Fundamentals of Chinese Medicine by the East Asian Medical Studies Society, Paradigm Publications, Brookline, MA, 1985. This is a more technical introduction and overview of Chinese medicine intended for professional entry level students.

Traditional Medicine in Contemporary China by Nathan Sivin, Center for Chinese Studies, University of Michigan, Ann Arbor, 1987. This book discusses the development of Chinese medicine in China in the last half century as well as introducing all the basic concepts of Chinese medical theory and practice.

Rooted in Spirit: The Heart of Chinese Medicine by Claude Larre & Elisabeth Rochat de la Vallée, trans. by Sarah Stang, Station Hill Press, NY, 1995. This book explains the central concepts of

155

Chinese medicine from a decidely spiritual point of view. Essentially, it is commentary on the eight chapter of the *Nei Jing Ling Shu (Inner Classic: Spiritual Pivot)*.

In the Footsteps of the Yellow Emperor: Tracing the History of Traditional Acupuncture by Peter Eckman, Cypress Book Company, San Francisco, 1996. This book is a history of Chinese medicine and especially acupuncture. In it, the author traces how acupuncture came to Europe and America from China, Hong Kong, Taiwan, Japan, and Korea in the early and middle part of this century. Included are nontechnical discussions of basic Chinese medical theory and concepts.

Knowing Practice: The Clinical Encounter of Chinese Medicine by Judith Farquhar, Westview Press, Boulder, CO, 1994. This book is a more scholarly approach to the recent history of Chinese medicine in the People's Republic of China as well as an introduction to the basic methodology of Chinese medical practice. Although written by an academic sinologist and not a practitioner, it nonetheless contains many insightful and perceptive observations on the differences between traditional Chinese and modern Western medicines.

Imperial Secrets of Health and Longevity by Bob Flaws, Blue Poppy Press, Inc., Boulder, CO, 1994. This book includes a section on Chinese dietary therapy and generally introduces the basic concepts of good health according to Chinese medicine.

Chinese Herbal Remedies by Albert Y. Leung, Universe Books, NY, 1984. This book is about simple Chinese herbal home remedies.
Legendary Chinese Healing Herbs by Henry C. Lu, Sterling Publishing, Inc., NY, 1991. This book is a fun way to begin learning about Chinese herbal medicine. It is full of interesting and entertaining anecdotes about Chinese medicinal herbs.

The Mystery of Longevity by Liu Zheng-cai, Foreign Languages Press, Beijing, 1990. This book is also about general principles and practice promoting good health according to Chinese medicine.

For more information on Chinese gynecology, see:

Curing PMSNaturally with Chinese Medicine by Bob Flaws, Blue Poppy Press, Boulder, CO, 1997. This book is an introduction to Chinese medical theory in terms of PMS written by one of the West's foremost practitioners of Chinese herbal medicine for nonprofessional women readers.

Menopause, A Second Spring: Make A Smooth Transition with Traditional Chinese Medicine by Honora Lee Wolfe, Blue Poppy Press, Boulder, CO, 1995. Written by the same author as the above book, this is a basic introduction to Chinese medicine and how it diagnoses and treats perimenopausal disorders, including osteoporosis.

Endometriosis, Infertility and Traditional Chinese Medicine by Bob Flaws, Blue Poppy Press, Boulder, CO, 1996. Similar to the above two books in conception and tone, this book deals with the Chinese medical diagnosis and treatment of endometriosis and infertility in an easy to understand way.

A Handbook of Menstrual Diseases in Chinese Medicine by Bob Flaws, Blue Poppy Press, Boulder, CO, 1997. This is a comprehensive professional clinical manual on the diagnosis and treatment of dozens of menstrual and premenstrual complaints with both Chinese herbal medicine and acupuncture.

A Handbook of Traditional Chinese Gynecology by the Zhejiang College of Chinese Medicine, Blue Poppy Press, Boulder, CO, 1995. This is also a professional clinical manual covering the diagnosis and treatment of menstrual diseases, abnormal vaginal discharge diseases, gestational and birthing diseases, postpartum diseases, and a number of so-called miscellaneous diseases, such as mastitis, uterine prolapse, and infertility.

Concise Traditional Chinese Gynecology by the Nanjing College of Chinese Medicine, Jiangsu Science & Technology Publishing House, Nanjing, 1988. This is a shorter, more condensed clinical manual on basic Chinese gynecology intended for professional readers.

The English-Chinese Encyclopedia of Practical Traditional Chinese Medicine, Gynecology by Xuan Jia-sheng *et al.*, Higher Education Press, Beijing, 1990. This is another professional entry level text on Chinese gynecology covering comparable material to the above two titles.

For more information on Chinese dietary therapy, see:

The Tao of Healthy Eating According to Traditional Chinese Medicine by Bob Flaws, Blue Poppy Press, Boulder, CO, 1997. This book is a layperson's primer on Chinese dietary therapy. It includes detailed sections on the clear, bland diet as well as sections on chronic candidiasis and allergies.

Prince Wen Hui's Cook: Chinese Dietary Therapy by Bob Flaws & Honora Lee Wolfe, Paradigm Publications, Brookline, MA, 1983. This book is an introduction to Chinese dietary therapy. Although some of the information it contains is dated, it does give the Chinese medicinal descriptions of most foods commonly eaten in the West.

The Book of Jook: Chinese Medicinal Porridges, A Healthy Alternative to the Typical Western Breakfast by Bob Flaws, Blue Poppy Press, Boulder, CO, 1995. This book is specifically about Chinese medicinal porridges made with very simple combinations of Chinese medicinal herbs.

The Tao of Nutrition by Maoshing Ni, Union of Tao and Man, Los Angeles, 1989

Harmony Rules: The Chinese Way of Health Through Food by Gary Butt & Frena Bloomfield, Samuel Weiser, Inc., York Beach, ME, 1985

Chinese System of Food Cures: Prevention & Remedies by Henry C. Lu, Sterling Publishing Co., Inc., NY, 1986

A Practical English-Chinese Library of Traditional Chinese Medicine: Chinese Medicated Diet ed. by Zhang En-qin, Shanghai College of Traditional Chinese Medicine Publishing House, Shanghai, 1990

Eating Your Way to Health—Dietotherapy in Traditional Chinese Medicine by Cai Jing-feng, Foreign Languages Press, Beijing, 1988

Chinese Medical Glossary

Chinese medicine is a system unto itself. Its technical terms are uniquely its own and cannot be reduced to the definitions of Western medicine without destroying the very fabric and logic of Chinese medicine. Ultimately, because Chinese medicine was created in the Chinese language, Chinese medicine is best and really only understood in that language. Nevertheless, as Westerners trying to understand Chinese medicine, we must translate the technical terms of Chinese medicine in English words. If some of these technical translations sound at first peculiar and their meaning is not immediately transparent, this is because no equivalent concepts exist in everyday English.

In the past, some Western authors have erroneously translated technical Chinese medical terms using Western medical or at least quasi-scientific words in an attempt to make this system more acceptable to Western audiences. For instance, the words tonify and sedate are commonly seen in the Western Chinese medical literature even though, in the case of sedate, its meaning is 180° opposite to the Chinese understanding of the word *xie*. *Xie* means to drain off something which has pooled and accumulated. That accumulation is seen as something excess which should not be lingering where it is. Because it is accumulating somewhere where it shouldn't, it is impeding and obstructing whatever should be moving to and through that area. The word sedate comes from the Latin word *sedere*, to sit. Therefore, the word sedate means to make something sit still. In English, we get the word sediment from this same root. However, the Chinese *xie* means draining off which is sitting somewhere erroneously. Therefore, to think that one is going to sedate what is already sitting is a great mistake in understanding the clinical implication and application of this technical term.

Therefore, in order to preserve the integrity of this system while still making it intelligible to English language readers, I have appended the following glossary of Chinese medical technical terms. The terms themselves are based on Nigel Wiseman's *English-Chinese Chinese-English Dictionary of Chinese Medicine* published by the Hunan Science & Technology Press in Changsha, Hunan, People's Republic of China in 1995. Dr. Wiseman is, I (Bob Flaws) believe, the greatest Western scholar in terms of the translation of Chinese medicine into English. As a Chinese reader myself, although I often find Wiseman's terms awkward sounding at first, I also think they convey most accurately the Chinese under-standing and logic of these terms.

Acquired essence: Essence manufactured out of the surplus of qi and blood in turn created out of the refined essence of food and drink

Acupoints: Those places on the channels and network vessels where qi and blood tend to collect in denser concentrations, and thus those places where the qi and blood in the channels are especially available for manipulation

Acupuncture: The regulation of qi flow by the stimulation of certain points located on the channels and network vessels achieved mainly by the insertion of fine needles into these points

Aromatherapy: Using various scents and smells to treat and prevent disease

Ascendant hyperactivity of liver yang: Upwardly out of control counterflow of liver yang due to insufficient yin to hold it down in the lower part of the body

Bedroom taxation: Fatigue or vacuity due to excessive sex

Blood: The red colored fluid which flows in the vessels and nourishes and constructs the tissues of the body

Blood stasis: Also called dead blood, malign blood, and dry blood, blood stasis is blood which is no longer moving through the vessels as it should. Instead it is precipitated in the vessels like silt in a river. Like silt, it then obstructs the free flow of the blood in the vessels and also impedes the production of new or fresh blood.

Blood vacuity: Insufficient blood manifesting in diminished nourishment, construction, and moistening of body tissues

Bowels: The hollow yang organs of Chinese medicine

Central qi: Also called the middle qi, this is synonymous with the spleen-stomach qi

Channels: The main routes for the distribution of qi and blood, but mainly qi

Chong & ren: Two of the eight extraordinary vessels which act as reservoirs for all the other channels and vessels of the body. These two govern women's menstruation, reproduction, and lactation in particular.

Clear: The pure or clear part of food and drink ingested which is then turned into qi and blood

Counterflow: An erroneous flow of qi, usually upward but sometimes horizontally as well

Damp heat: A combination of accumulated dampness mixed with pathological heat often associated with sores, abnormal vaginal discharges, and some types of menstrual and body pain

Dampness: A pathological accumulation of body fluids

Decoction: A method of administering Chinese medicinals by boiling these medicinals in water, removing the dregs, and drinking the resulting medicinal liquid

Depression: Stagnation and lack of movement, as in liver depression qi stagnation

Depressive heat: Heat due to enduring or severe qi stagnation which then transforms into heat

Drain: To drain off or away some pathological qi or substance from where it is replete or excess

Essence: A stored, very potent form of substance and qi, usually yin when compared to yang qi, but can be transformed into yang qi

163

Five phase theory: A ancient Chinese system of correspondences dividing up all of reality into five phases of development which then mutually engender and check each other according to definite sequences

Heat toxins: A particularly virulent and concentrated type of pathological heat often associated with purulence (*i.e.*, pus formation), sores, and sometimes, but not always, malignancies

Heliotherapy: Exposure of the body to sunlight in order to treat and prevent disease

Hydrotherapy: Using various baths and water applications to treat and prevent disease

Lassitude of the spirit: A listless or apathetic affect or emotional demeanor due to obvious fatigue of the mind and body

Life gate fire: Another name for kidney yang or kidney fire, seen as the ultimate source of yang qi in the body

Magnet therapy: Applying magnets to acupuncture points to treat and prevent disease

Moxibustion: Burning the herb Artemisia Argyium on, over, or near acupuncture points in order to add yang qi, warm cold, or promote the movement of the qi and blood

Network vessels: Small vessels which form a net-like web insuring the flow of qi and blood to all body tissues

Phlegm: A pathological accumulation of phlegm or mucus congealed from dampness or body fluids

Qi: Activity, function, that which moves, transforms, defends, restrains, and warms

Portals: Also called orifices, the openings of the sensory organs and the opening of the heart through which the spirit makes contact with the world outside

Qi mechanism: The process of transforming yin substance controlled and promoted by the qi, largely synonymous with the process of digestion

Qi vacuity: Insufficient qi manifesting in diminished movement, transformation, and function

Repletion: Excess or fullness, almost always pathological

164

Seven star hammer: A small hammer with needles embedded in its head used to stimulate acupoints without actually inserting needles

Spirit: The accumulation of qi in the heart which manifests as consciousness, sensory awareness, and mental-emotional function

Stagnation: Non-movement of the qi, lack of free flow, constraint

Supplement: To add to or augment, as in supplementing the qi, blood, yin, or yang

Turbid: The yin, impure, turbid part of food and drink which is sent downward to be excreted as waste

Vacuity: Emptiness or insufficiency, typically of qi, blood, yin, or yang

Vacuity cold: Obvious signs and symptoms of cold due to a lack or insufficiency of yang qi

Vacuity heat: Heat due to hyperactive yang in turn due to insufficient controlling yin

Vessels: The main routes for the distribution of qi and blood, but mainly blood

Viscera: The sold yin organs of Chinese medicine

Yin: In the body, substance and nourishment

Yin vacuity: Insufficient yin substance necessary to both nourish, control, and counterbalance yang activity

Yang: In the body, function, movement, activity, transformation

Yang vacuity: Insufficient warming and transforming function giving rise to symptoms of cold in the body

Breast Self-exam

Despite continual educational articles in women's magazines, pamphlets circulated by women's health clinics, and admonitions from all types of health care practitioners, the majority of women do not do regular breast self-exams. This fact is due to two main reasons. First, many women are concerned that they lack the ability to examine themselves correctly or effectively and, more importantly, they are afraid to search for something they do not want to find. Recently, a new method of breast self-examination called MammaCare has been promulgated by a number of breast cancer research and health organizations. This method has women examine a larger area than other methods—from the collorbone down to the bra line and farom the underarm across to the breast bone. The emphasis here is on the upper, outer breast quadrant, where nearly 50% of breast tumors develop. It also prescribes a verticle search pattern with three types of finger pressure—light, medium, and deep— which helps identify tumors at various depths in the breast tissue.

There has been a research study confirming the increased effectiveness of the MammaCare method done by Dr. Suzanne Fletcher, a professor of ambulatory and preventive medicine at Harvard.[55] In her study, women were divided into three groups: the first received MammCare training, the second taught the more traditional breast self-exam, and the third received no training at all. A year later, the MammaCare group had detected tumors significantly better than the other groups.

---

[55] Castleman, Michael, *Family Circle, op.cit.*, p. 66

The MammaCare method can be learned at home with the MammaCare Personal Learning System, which includes an instructional video and booklet, and a breast model containing simulated benign and potentially cancerous lumps for $69.50. For information call Mammtech Corp at 1-800-MAM-CARE or write PO Box 15748, Gainesville, FL 32604.

Brassieres & Breast Health

There have been research studies in recent years that suggest that wearing a bra for more than a certain number of hours per day can increase your risk for breast cancer.[56] Other studies say this is baloney. From a Chinese medical point of view, there is a certain amount of logic to the idea that anything which constricts the breast tissue can impede the flow of qi and blood through the breast. On the other hand, this can become very crazy making.

Personally, I (Honora Lee Wolfe) have chosen a middle path with bras that works for me. I wear them if the clothes I am wearing will look better with a bra, or if I am simply in the mood to wear one. However, I try to take it off at the end of the work day, if that is convenient or possible. On days where I am not working or I am just going to be in front of my personal computer, I often choose fitted tank tops or camisoles for modesty and comfort, but which do not constrict my breasts and which fit comfortably under most clothes. I have found that catalogs such as Winter Silks (800-648-7455), Victoria's Secret (800-888-8200), Decent Exposures (800-505-4949), Title Nine Sports (800-609-0092), and Seventh Generation (800-869-3446) carry a variety of products that work very nicely for these purposes.

Women have many different relationships with bras. Some women get rashes from wearing them. Many women are uncomfortable without them for either physical or emotional reasons. Many women find them sexy and feminine or like to use them as part of lovemaking. Some women think of them almost like a

---

[56] Ross-Singer, Sydney and Grismaijer, Sonia, "Dressed to Kill: The Link Between Breast Cancer & Bras, *Skeptical Inquirer*, Nov.-Dec., 1995, Vol. 19, #6, p. 13-14.

form of jewelry or adornment and some think of them as a prison. Women with fibrocystic breast discomfort often find the support of a bra is soothing during days that the breasts are sore or distended.

Given that studies about wearing a bra and cancer risk are very preliminary and that all women have some cancer risk factors, it seems appropriate to try and cultivate some moderation about whether, how often, and what type of bras or other breast support you choose. These are very personal choices and it seems to me not to be useful to make oneself neurotic about them. We are lucky that there is such a variety of underwear options available from which modern women can choose and still be as comfortable, modest, and/or sexy as she likes.

General Index

A

abdominal distention after meals 59
abdominal massage 89, 90
abortion, artificial 66
acne 58, 62
acne, premenstrual 58
acupuncture 56, 70, 71, 78, 88, 94, 96, 100, 116-118, 120-122, 135, 149-151, 155-157, 162, 164
agitation 23, 60, 144
allergies, sinusitis 61
anger 25, 29, 30, 32, 42, 58, 65, 67, 72, 119, 136, 140, 141, 144, 145
anger, suppressed 29, 67
appetite, reduced or loss of 32, 59
aromatherapy 98-100, 162
aspiration 1, 9, 13, 15
asthma 28, 60

B

bleeding, pathological 31
bloating after meals 32, 128
blood, insufficient 38, 51, 169
breast cancer 1-3, 7, 10-15, 44, 47, 56, 63-70, 82, 85, 115, 121, 167, 169
breast distention and pain 7, 40, 41, 44-48, 51, 57, 96, 108, 118, 119, 136-139, 142, 144
breast feeding 11, 66
breast feeding, improper 66
breast malignancies 2, 12
breast pain and distention, 29
breast rock 65, 66
breast self-examination 6, 14, 163
breasts, swollen 1, 112

C

cancer, breast 1-3, 7, 10-15, 44, 47, 56, 63-70, 82, 85, 115, 121, 167, 169
cancer, prostate 13
canker sores, mouth or 32
chest oppression 60, 136-139

Chinese herbal medicine 70, 113-115, 122-125, 135, 155-157
chocolate 81, 83, 84
coffee 83, 84, 86, 88, 99
cough, chronic 27
craving for sweets 59
crying, easy 58, 59

D

dandelion 104-107, 111
digestive disturbance, chronic 29
disc disease, degenerative 28
dizziness 56, 60, 79, 129, 137, 138, 144, 146
dream-disturbed sleep 60
drug use 27
dryness, excessive 27
dysmenorrhea 58

E

ear acupuncture 88, 122
ears, ringing in the 27
edema 27
edematous swelling 59
emotional stress 48, 51, 66, 139
emotional symptoms 29
environmental and chemical pollutants 68
estrogen/progesterone imbalance 9
estrogen, excessive 7
exercise, too little 52
extremities, tingling and numbness in the 32
eye problems 30

F

face and hands, brown spots on the 61
facial color sallow white 146
fatigue 59, 60, 62, 79, 83, 102, 103, 115, 119, 121, 129, 131, 140, 162, 164
fear, constant or excessive 28
feet, cold 60, 62

171

PMS 1, 7, 8, 29, 40, 41-51, 63, 71, 81, 104, 119, 122, 125, 157
pollutants, environmental and chemical 66
porridges 106, 158
pregnancy, early terminated 66
premenstrual acne 58
premenstrual low back pain 62
professional therapies 113
prostate cancer 13
pus or purulence 62
qi stagnation 29, 43-45, 51-53, 57, 58, 60, 61, 63, 67, 69, 70, 72, 75, 80, 83-85, 86, 96, 98, 100, 109, 119, 121, 126, 132, 142, 145, 147, 148, 163
research, outcome-based 135

S

self-image 2
self-massage 89, 90, 92-95
sex drive, decreased 60, 62
sexual activity, excessive 27
sighing, frequent 57
sinusitis, allergies 60
sleep, dream-disturbed 60
sores or ulcers, open 62
stools, loose 55, 59, 62, 79, 102, 103, 109, 119-121, 128, 146
stress/frustration, unrelieved 57
sweets, craving for 57
swelling, localized 62

T

teas, medicinal 86, 106
thermography 13
thread moxibustion 101
tingling and numbness in the extremities 32
tinnitus 60, 138

U, V, W, X

ultrasonography 13
urination, nighttime 27, 62, 102, 103
varicose veins 61

vertigo 144, 146
weeping, bitter 66
weight gain 62
worry and anger 65
xanthines 83

OTHER BOOKS ON CHINESE MEDICINE AVAILABLE FROM BLUE POPPY PRESS

3450 Penrose Place, Suite 110, Boulder, CO 80301
For ordering 1-800-487-9296 PH. 303\447-8372 FAX 303\447-0740

A NEW AMERICAN ACUPUNC-TURE by Mark Seem, ISBN 0-936185-44-9

ACUPOINT POCKET REFERENCE ISBN 0-936185-93-7

ACUPUNCTURE AND MOXI-BUSTION FORMULAS & TREATMENTS by Cheng Dan-an, trans. by Wu Ming, ISBN 0-936185-68-6

ACUTE ABDOMINAL SYN-DROMES: Their Diagnosis & Treatment by Combined Chinese-Western Medicine by Alon Marcus, ISBN 0-936185-31-7

AGING & BLOOD STASIS: A New Approach to TCM Geriatrics by Yan De-xin, ISBN 0-936185-63-5

AIDS & ITS TREATMENT ACCORDING TO TRADITIONAL CHINESE MEDICINE by Huang Bing-shan, trans. by Fu-Di & Bob Flaws, ISBN 0-936185-28-7

THE BOOK OF JOOK: Chinese Medicinal Porridges, An Alterna-tive to the Typical Western Break-fast by B. Flaws, ISBN0-936185-60-0

CHINESE MEDICAL PALMIS-TRY: Your Health in Your Hand by Zong Xiao-fan & Gary Liscum, ISBN 0-936185-64-3

CHINESE MEDICINAL TEAS: Simple, Proven, Folk Formulas for Common Diseases & Promoting Health by Zong Xiao-fan & Gary Liscum, ISBN 0-936185-76-7

CHINESE MEDICINAL WINES & ELIXIRS by Bob Flaws, ISBN 0-936185-58-9

CHINESE PEDIATRIC MAS-SAGE THERAPY: *A Parent's & Practitioner's Guide to the Prevention & Treatment of Childhood Illness* by Fan Ya-li, ISBN 0-936185-54-6

CHINESE SELF-MASSAGE THE-RAPY: The Easy Way to Health by Fan Ya-li ISBN 0-936185-74-0

CLASSICAL MOXIBUSTION SKILLS in Clinical Practice by Sung Baek, ISBN 0-936185-16-3

A COMPENDIUM OF TCM PAT-TERNS & TREATMENTS by Bob Flaws & Daniel Finney, ISBN 0-936185-70-8

CURING ARTHRITIS NATURALLY WITH CHINESE MEDICINE by Douglas Frank & Bob Flaws ISBN 0-936185-87-2

CURING HAY FEVER NATURALLY WITH CHINESE MEDICINE by Bob Flaws, ISBN 0-936185-91-0

CURING INSOMNIA NATURALLY WITH CHINESE MEDICINE by Bob Flaws ISBN 0-936185-85-6

CURING PMS NATURALLY WITH CHINESE MEDICINE by Bob Flaws ISBN 0-936185-85-6

THE DAO OF INCREASING LONGEVITY AND CONSERVING ONE'S LIFE by Anna Lin & Bob Flaws, ISBN 0-936185-24-4

THE DAO OF HEALTHY EATING ACCORDING TO CHINESE MEDICINE by Bob Flaws, ISBN 0-936185-92-9

THE DIVINE FARMER'S MATERIA MEDICA (*A Translation of the Shen Nong Ben Cao*) by Yang Shou-zhong ISBN 0-936185-96-1

THE DIVINELY RESPONDING CLASSIC: *A Translation of the Shen Ying Jing from Zhen Jiu Da Cheng*, trans. by Yang Shou-zhong & Liu Feng-ting ISBN 0-936185-55-4

DUI YAO: THE ART OF COMBINING CHINESE HERBAL MEDICINALS by Philippe Sionneau ISBN 0-936185-81-3

ENDOMETRIOSIS, INFERTILITY AND TRADITIONAL CHINESE MEDICINE: A Laywoman's Guide by Bob Flaws ISBN 0-936185-14-7

EXTRA TREATISES BASED ON INVESTIGATION & INQUIRY: *A Translation of Zhu Dan-xi's Ge Zhi Yu Lun*, by Yang Shou-zhong & Duan Wu-jin, ISBN 0-936185-53-8

FIRE IN THE VALLEY: TCM Diagnosis & Treatment of Vaginal Diseases ISBN 0-936185-25-2

FLESHING OUT THE BONES: The Importance of Case Histories in Chin. Med. trans. by Chip Chace. ISBN 0-936185-30-9

FU QING-ZHU'S GYNECOLOGY trans. by Yang Shou-zhong and Liu Da-wei, ISBN 0-936185-35-X

FULFILLING THE ESSENCE: A *Handbook of Traditional & Contemporary Treatments for Female Infertility* by Bob Flaws, ISBN 0-936185-48-1

GOLDEN NEEDLE WANG LE-TING: A 20th Century Master's Approach to Acupuncture by Yu Hui-chan and Han Fu-ru, trans. by Shuai Xue-zhong,

A HANDBOOK OF TRADITIONAL CHINESE DERMATOLOGY by Liang Jian-hui, trans. by Zhang & Flaws, ISBN 0-936185-07-4

A HANDBOOK OF TRADITIONAL CHINESE GYNECOLOGY by Zhejiang College of TCM, trans. by Zhang Ting-liang, ISBN 0-936185-06-6 (4th edit.)

A HANDBOOK OF MENSTRUAL DISEASES IN CHINESE MEDICINE by Bob Flaws ISBN 0-936185-82-1

A HANDBOOK of TCM PEDIATRICS by Bob Flaws, ISBN 0-936185-72-4

A HANDBOOK OF TCM UROLOGY & MALE SEXUAL DYSFUNCTION by Anna Lin, OMD, ISBN 0-936185-36-8

THE HEART & ESSENCE OF DAN-XI'S METHODS OF TREATMENT by Xu Dan-xi, trans. by Yang, ISBN 0-926185-49-X

THE HEART TRANSMISSION OF MEDICINE by Liu Yi-ren, trans. by Yang Shou-zhong ISBN 0-936185-83-X

HIGHLIGHTS OF ANCIENT ACUPUNCTURE PRESCRIPTIONS trans. by Wolfe & Crescenz ISBN 0-936185-23-6

How to Have A HEALTHY PREGNANCY, HEALTHY BIRTH with Chinese Medicine by Honora Lee Wolfe, ISBN 0-936185-40-6

THE SYSTEMATIC CLASSIC OF ACUPUNCTURE & MOXIBUS-TION (*Jia Yi Jing*) by Huang-fu Mi, trans. by Yang Shou-zhong & Charles Chace, ISBN 0-936185-29-5

THE TREATMENT OF DISEASE IN TCM, Vol I: Diseases of the Head & Face Including Mental/Emotional Disorders by Philippe Sionneau & Lü Gang, ISBN 0-936185-69-4

THE TREATMENT OF DISEASE IN TCM, Vol. II: Diseases of the Eyes, Ears, Nose, & Throat by Sionneau & Lü, ISBN 0-936185-69-4

THE TREATMENT OF DISEASE, VOL. III: Diseases of the Mouth, Lips, Tongue, Teeth & Gums, by Sionneau & Lü, ISBN 0-936185-79-1

THE TREATMENT OF DISEASE, VOL VI: Diseases of the Neck, Shoulders, Upper & Lower Back, & Extremities, by Philippe Sionneau & Lü Gang, ISBN 0-936185-89-9

THE TREATMENT OF EXTERNAL DISEASES WITH ACUPUNCTURE & MOXIBUSTION by Yan Cui-lan and Zhu Yun-long, ISBN 0-936185-80-5